HEALTHY BY DESIGN

THE BREAKTHROUGH METHOD

Your Guided Path to Weight Loss, God's Way

CATHY MORENZIE

+ 11 Leaders in Health & Weight Loss

Published: March 19, 2024

ISBN: 9781990078224 (print)

9781990078231 (digital)

Published by Guiding Light Publishing
46 Bell St, Barrie, ON, Canada, L4N 0H9

Note: The information in this book is for educational purposes only and is not recommended as a means of diagnosing or treating illness. All situations concerning physical or mental health should be supervised by a health professional knowledgeable in treating that particular condition. Neither the author nor anyone affiliated with Healthy by Design dispenses medical advice, nor do they prescribe any remedies or assume any responsibility for anyone who chooses to treat themselves.

Cover photo by T. Preston Squire

Cover design by Kim Monteforte kimmontefortebookdesign.com

Interior design by Daria Lacy

What people are saying about The Breakthrough Method

"Cathy is more than a weight loss coach; she is a freedom coach who values transparency and identifying the root causes of weight loss cycles. Whether you are just starting, starting again, or continuing the journey, The Breakthrough Method invites you to experience your next level of freedom! Within the pages of this book, Cathy expertly guides you through the process that will empower you to achieve your goals and transform your entire being."

Sharon Roshell Thomas | Host of The Authenticated Life Podcast

"Cathy Morenzie provides powerful insight into the relationship between our body, mind and spirit. She gives practical strategies to develop both healthy mindsets and strong bodies. This is the most well rounded approach to weight loss that I have ever read."

Melody Dowlearn | CEO & Founder of The Identity Academy and author of the bestselling book *Kingdom Identity*

"This book delivers a 2-in-1 benefit. Any reader who applies these principles will discover that their faith and connection to God have skyrocketed in addition to the bodily benefits they were initially seeking. It shows how to cleanse the inner vessel so the outer vessel shines for the Lord (and ourselves). The author's deep understanding of the Bible shines through every page, not to mention her present joy and enthusiasm for God. The writing style is a delight--consummately clear, empathetic, faith-promoting, and actionable. It's impossible to read without feeling uplifted and enticed to apply the wise blend of biblical and science-based health principles. For readers whose walk with Jesus is important to them, this is THE book to help you honor God in heart, soul, and body like never before."

R. Christian Bohlen | Author of *Jesus Christ, His Life and Mine* | *Healing the Stormy Marriage*

"Cathy's Breakthrough Method is a must-read for anyone seeking a wholistic God-centered approach to better health and freedom from the bondage of excess weight. Not only does this book bridge the gap between our physical bodies and spiritual well-being but it also provides practical, God-centered principles for achieving lasting health, unlike traditional quick-fix models. The Breakthrough Method, compassionately outlined in these pages, guides you through a journey of self-discovery, helping you align your health goals with God's purpose for your life. It introduces new and refreshing concepts such as energy management and emotional resilience. Each powerful principle will shine a new light on the truth about losing weight. Cathy truly challenges the diet plan mentality, changes your perspective, and gives a clear roadmap to a healthier, more fulfilling life."

Inger Wyatt | Executive Pastor, Speaking Spirit
Ministries - Richmond, Virginia

Contents

My Personal Story

What do you see when you look in the mirror? Do you see more than just your reflection? Do you see the years of struggle, the countless battles fought in the quiet of your mind, and the relentless pursuit of an unattainable ideal?

For years, I looked in the mirror and saw only flaws. Each morning, I stood before that unforgiving glass, my gaze fixated on every perceived imperfection. The harsh bathroom light seemed to illuminate my self-doubt, casting long shadows on my self-worth. I was enslaved in an unending cycle of self-criticism, convinced that the number on the scale and the reflection that stared back at me in the mirror held the key to my happiness and self-worth.

I was not alone in this struggle. As I shared my personal challenges in my previous *Healthy by Design* books, I realized that, like countless other women around the world, I was caught in the relentless web of diets, weight loss programs, and the unending pursuit of an idealized image. Even though I was an advocate for good health and wellness, I secretly measured my worth in pounds and ounces, and my reflection in the mirror became a cruel judge of my value. I believed that my self-esteem was directly proportional to the number that blinked back at me from the scale.

As far back as I can remember, I used to always be on a diet. The world had ingrained in me the harmful notion that beauty could be distilled into a dress size, a waist measurement, or a number on the scale. I had internalized this toxic narrative to the point where it guided the choices I made about my life and my body.

I remember the pivotal moment when the opportunity arose for me to attend a school far away from home. In selecting my courses, physical education was the obvious choice. It was, in my mind, the most direct path toward achieving my elusive goal of attaining the ideal body. I believed that if I could just mold my physical form to match the standards imposed by society, I would finally be deemed beautiful and worthy of love and acceptance.

Little did I know that this journey, though arduous, would eventually lead me to a place of introspection and discovery. It was a journey that took me far beyond focusing on my physical body, forcing me to confront the deep-seated beliefs and damaging narratives that had held me captive for so long.

The pursuit of that idealized image would ultimately serve as the catalyst for a remarkable shift in my life—a shift that would not only change the way I perceived myself but would also set me on a path to help others break free from the shackles of the diet mindset. Part of my freedom allowed me to come to the understanding that this journey has no final destination. The joy is in the journey itself. It's the lessons I learned and continue to learn, the fruits I'm cultivating such as discipline, self-control, long-suffering and patience, that are transforming me from the inside out. It's the journey to my countless breakthroughs in the journey that free me day by day, little by little, and it will do the same for you, too.

This book, *The Breakthrough Method*, is not just about losing weight or following another diet plan. It's about breaking free from the chains of a diet mindset and embracing a journey of holistic health—a journey that goes deeper than the superficial goals we often set for ourselves.

As Christian women we are called to live abundantly, to honor and steward the temples that house our souls. Our faith teaches us that God does not look at the outward appearance but at the heart (1 Samuel 16:7). So, it's time we shift our focus and embark on a transformative journey that encompasses mind, body, and spirit.

In the chapters that follow, we will explore the fourteen crucial paradigm shifts necessary to break the chains of the diet mindset and embrace a new path to holistic health. These shifts not only form the foundation for my coaching practice but also represent the very same principles that all of our

Weight Loss God's Way coaches are trained in. This method you're about to learn is what gets results for our clients.

At the end of this book, you will have the privilege of meeting eleven of these extraordinary coaches—women who have their own stories to tell, their own struggles to share, and their unique insights into faith and health. Their experiences will serve as beacons of hope, guiding you toward a brighter, healthier, and more spiritually connected future.

As we journey together I invite you to reflect on your own life, your own struggles, and the narratives that have shaped your perception of yourself. Are you ready to break free from the reflection trap and discover a new way of living—one that honors your body as a sacred vessel of God's grace and values your worth beyond the superficial standards of the world?

Join me on this journey, dear sisters, as we transform not only the way you approach your health but also the way you see yourself in the eyes of the One who created you.

Are you ready to break free from the diet mindset and embrace a path of holistic health? Are you ready for your breakthrough?

Introduction

I am absolutely delighted that you've chosen to embark on this transformative journey as we explore the pages of this book together.

I want you to know that I consider your trust in me a sacred responsibility, and I wholeheartedly commit to sharing not only my thirty-five years of experience in the health and weight loss industry but also the Holy Spirit-inspired insights that have guided me. Together, we will explore the path to achieving your healthy weight, strengthening your faith, and healing past wounds that may have kept you trapped in the cycle of yo-yo dieting.

The journey that culminated in this book has been years in the making, stemming from the Breakthrough online course I've been privileged to teach since 2015. This course has empowered women to shed weight, fortify their faith and mend the wounds of their past, liberating them from the burdens of relentless dieting while achieving their healthy weight. With this book my aim is to share a portion of the life-altering wisdom from the course with a broader audience, reaching those who may never have the chance to participate in our programs, whether online or in person.

My earnest hope and prayer for you is that *The Breakthrough Method* will revolutionize the way you approach your health, weight, and life's challenges. Rest assured that every valley you've traversed will now serve as a stepping stone toward your future aspirations.

I invite you to reflect on those valleys—perhaps you can recall one, or maybe ten of them. Know this: these valleys are the bedrock for your breakthrough. One of our coaches, Gail, taught me that most fertile soil is often found in the valleys. It's here that rain and snowmelt flow down from the mountains, leaving behind rich deposits of organic sediments and nutrients in the valleys below. And in my own health journey, I know this to be true.

These valleys have been my crucible for growth, revealing the truth of who I am and to Whom I belong. Through these experiences, I've come to understand my identity in Christ. I've learned and continue to learn how to transform my relationship with food, my body, my health, exercise, and God. Exercise is no longer a form of punishment but an act of worship. Food is no longer a reward or a source of comfort but a powerful form of medicine and a divine gift. My health is cherished as one of my greatest assets. My body is no longer objectified, but revered as the temple housing the living God. God Himself is no longer a distant, judgmental figure but a loving, compassionate Father who knows me intimately.

This is what I mean by breakthrough—it's not a single, isolated event but a continuous journey of transformation. It's a process that I'm excited to guide you through, sharing the blessings and insights I've gained along the way.

The Breakthrough Method will:

- Reframe your entire perspective about what it means to lose weight and help you shed the diet mentality (Romans 12:2)

- Provide you with a practical blueprint that you can start implementing right now (1 Corinthians 9:26)

- Address every aspect of your being—spirit, soul, and body (1 Thessalonians 5:23)

- Teach you how to let go and release your grip on dieting (1 Peter 5:7)

- Facilitate change from the inside out (Psalms 138:3)

- Tackle the root causes of overeating and self sabotaging your health

- Ground your desire to release weight in something deeper than just the number on the scale

- Heal your unhealthy relationship with food and your body

- Illuminate why this journey has felt so challenging in the past

- Show you how to apply faith and action to your weight releasing journey

- Provide you with a plan to keep moving forward even when the odds seem stacked against you

- Help you anchor your health in your identity in Christ

That's what makes this book so different. Each page will invite you to keep showing up for the process with love and compassion while gently peeling back the layers that have brought you to this juncture in your health. Let this be the turning point in your life. As you set out to get healthier, this journey will take you to depths you never imagined, transforming not only your health but also your faith if you allow it to.

Breakthrough is not an event or a goal. It is a way of life.

Before we get started, let me offer a personal disclaimer. As I wrote this book, it became abundantly clear to me that I am offering a theological perspective on weight releasing from a Biblical standpoint. This view supplements the basic principles of physiology and nutrition and is by no means a replacement for good old-fashioned effort. My hope is that what you read will inspire you to make healthier food choices and become more active. If you seek specific guidance on nutrition and exercise, please refer to my other books.

Why the word 'Breakthrough'?

In the Biblical sense, breakthrough can be defined as a period in the life of a believer when they gain a deeper understanding into God's truth, hear a clear word from the Lord that has a dramatic impact on their life, receive answer to prayer, or are finally released from a besetting sin that has been holding them back for a long time.

With this definition in mind you can raise your expectation to receive one, two, or all of the above outcomes after reading this book in the area of your health as well as other areas of your life.

In the process of breakthrough, God is teaching us to stop tenaciously clinging to the things we desperately want so badly—like achieving a certain number on the scale. He wants us to find our rest in Him and stop resisting the process. He wants us to release our grip on everything and trust Him for the outcome.

Breakthrough in the Bible

The Bible highlights many spiritual breakthroughs. The first one we'll study is from an unlikely character in the Bible, a man named Jacob.

Jacob's Breakthrough

Jacob, the father of the 12 tribes of Israel, is one of the most significant characters in the Old Testament. His name means, "he grasps the heel" or "he deceives", given to him because he struggled in the womb with his twin brother Esau by grabbing his heel.

Later on, when the twins were older, Jacob co-conspired with his mother to deceive his father in order to receive the blessing or birthright that should have gone to his older brother, Esau. (Gen 25:29-34). This spirit of deceit and trickery continued to plague Jacob throughout his life.

Like Jacob, many of us have also inherited deceitful or some other type of spirits from our parents or parents' parents (others include lying, pride, infirmity, addiction, anxiety, fear, abandonment). Or we may have acquired a hereditary illness such as diabetes, hypertension or high blood sugar. If we're not proactive and vigilant, they can keep us from attaining all that God has for us.

Thank God He has a greater inheritance waiting for us. He wants to show us that our past does not need to be our future if we confront it, overpower it, and reclaim our identity in Him. That's what God wanted for Jacob, and that's what God wants for us, too.

Let's pick up with the events that led to Jacob's breakthrough where we find him desperate, discouraged, and in despair—the fruits of a life lived in deceit. After fourteen years of being on the run, he decided to return home to confront his brother who he tricked out of his inheritance and birthright. (Genesis 27)

The scene is set in the middle of a desert where he is all alone, contemplating the anticipated ill-fated reunion with his brother who he deceived. At this lowest point, God showed up in the form of a man and wrestled with him all night.

> "So Jacob was left alone, and a man wrestled with him till daybreak. When the man saw that he could not overpower him, he touched the socket of Jacob's hip so that his hip was wrenched as he wrestled with the man.
>
> "Then the man said, 'Let me go, for it is daybreak.' But Jacob replied, 'I will not let you go unless you bless me.' The man asked him, 'What is your name?' 'Jacob,' he answered. Then the man said, 'Your name will no longer be Jacob, but Israel, because you have struggled with God and with men and have overcome.'
>
> "Jacob said, 'Please tell me your name.' But he replied, 'Why do you ask my name?' Then he blessed him there.
>
> "So Jacob called the place Peniel, saying, 'It is because I saw God face to face, and yet my life was spared.' The sun rose above him as he passed Peniel, and he was limping because of his hip." (Genesis 32:24-31 NIV)

Jacob sensed his opportunity for a breakthrough, so he latched on to the man and refused to let go. Are you ready to latch on and not let go until you receive your blessing? It will take some wrestling. My sister, refuse to let go of God until you receive your blessing. Refuse to settle until you see the face of God and are confident in the fact that your victory is at hand because you've spent time with Him.

Let your "limp" be your sign to the world that you've been with God. Let your limp be a reminder to yourself that God is your strength and you will forever need Him to walk a straight and sure path. Let your 'limp' signify your strong character that you've developed as a result of your struggle.

Paul's Breakthrough

Now we'll turn to one of the most important characters in the New Testament, the Apostle Paul. He is credited with shaping the history of Christianity.

Paul was a very religious Jew who was zealous in the persecution of Christians because he believed that they were a danger to the Jewish faith. In his zeal, Paul went to the high priest and requested permission to leave Jerusalem and travel 150 miles to Damascus, Syria to capture Christians who were fleeing persecution (Acts 9:1-2).

Fortunately, God had other plans for Paul (then called Saul) on that fateful trek to Damascus. This was the moment of Paul's breakthrough.

The InterVarsity Press commentary states that, "The most important event in human history apart from the life, death and resurrection of Jesus of Nazareth is the conversion to Christianity of Saul of Tarsus." That's a pretty big claim!! Saul's breakthrough is described as one of the most important events in human history!

> *"As he neared Damascus on his journey, suddenly a light from heaven flashed around him. He fell to the ground and heard a voice say to him, "Saul, Saul, why do you persecute me?"*
>
> *"Who are you, Lord?" Saul asked.*
>
> *"I am Jesus, whom you are persecuting," he replied. "Now get up and go into the city, and you will be told what you must do."*
>
> *The men traveling with Saul stood there speechless; they heard the sound but did not see anyone. Saul got up from the ground, but when he opened his eyes he could see nothing. So they led him by the hand into Damascus." (Acts 9:3-5 NIV)*

Once Paul was filled with the Holy Spirit and his sight returned, he redirected that same passion and zeal to preaching about Jesus in the synagogues. The Bible says that all who heard him were amazed (Acts 9:21). Can you imagine, one day you're murdering Christians and the next day you're the main spokesperson for the same cause you were condemning! Talk about a 180-degree turnaround. But the transformation had to be so dramatic and unbelievable that both Christians and Jews knew that it could only be God.

Like Jacob, Paul had a personal encounter with God that changed his life forever.

Paul's story teaches us that only God can make the impossible possible, that God will use our past sins so that we may serve him in the future. And lastly, that there is no sin too deep or conviction so strong that God can't fix. Maybe you've been overweight all your life. Maybe you've had an endless history of abusing food. Maybe you can't imagine ever giving up sugar or finding the desire to exercise. Let Paul's transformation remind you that God can meet you wherever you're at and turn your situation around from dire and impossible to possible.

> *"And we know that God causes everything to work together for the good of those who love God and are called according to his purpose for them." (Romans 8:28 NLT)*

Lydia's Breakthrough

Lastly let's look at a woman in the Bible to study our last example of breakthrough. Though we don't know as much about her as we do about Paul and Jacob, her breakthrough is no less significant. In fact, her immediate response to her encounter with God is a perfect depiction of how we can respond when we wholeheartedly allow God into our lives.

The Bible says that Lydia was a business woman who dealt in fine purple cloth (Acts 16:14). She is credited with being Paul's first European convert. Her breakthrough is significant because of her swift inward and outward response to Christ's call. As her heart was open she quickly responded by not only getting baptized but sharing this incredible gift by having her entire family also baptized. The truth of God's message always demands a response. It demands repentance. It demands trust in the finished work of Christ. It demands a life of discipleship, all of which became possible after her encounter.

The Scripture tells us that the Lord opened Lydia's heart (Acts 16:14). She did not do it in her own strength; it was not because of Paul's incredible preaching—it was the Lord Himself who did it. Just like the conversion stories of Paul and Jacob, it was the Lord who moved in her life to transform her. We learn again that God rewards those who diligently seek Him. Despite her offering prayer and meeting with women on the Sabbath day to offer worship to God, for some reason her heart was still closed. Sound familiar? We may love the Lord with all our heart, we may think we're saying all the right things and going through all the right motions, yet there's still something in us that keeps our hearts closed. Like Lydia, honestly seek the Lord and allow Him to open your heart. Ask Him to search you and show the areas of your life where you may be closed (Psalm 139:23).

Like Jacob, do you find yourself in a divine wrestling match with God, begging, pleading and constantly crying out to Him, only to try to overpower Him again with your self-will? Like Paul, are you passionate and driven, but for the wrong things?

Like Lydia, do you love the Lord, but for some reason your heart is closed? When you experience your breakthrough, will you be willing to bring your entire family along with you?

I understand the fear and frustration you feel as you desperately seek to change your life. I understand the fear of letting go and letting God be Lord over your health and your life. The freedom, peace, and joy that Jacob, Paul, and Lydia experienced are also available to you when you give yourself wholeheartedly to Him.

As it was with Jacob, Paul, and Lydia, so it will be with you. As you wrestle with God's spiritual truths, understand who you are in Christ, learn about His undying love for you, and you, too, will achieve your Breakthrough. As God touches you, changes you from the inside out and blesses you, you will learn to trust Him with every fiber of your being. Are you ready for God to move in your life? Get ready. It's your turn!

Principle #1: Create Clarity

The Truth You Must Face

Welcome to the first step in your health and weight-releasing journey—a journey that requires a delicate balance of honesty and introspection coupled with a generous dose of grace and self-compassion. Brace yourself, for we're about to dispel many myths and confront many truths that must be acknowledged to set your breakthrough in motion.

I'm an avid hiker. That's my thing. My goal is to hike the Bruce Trail in my lifetime. The Bruce Trail is approximately 900 kilometers (560 miles) long, making it one of Canada's longest continuous footpaths. It extends through the Niagara Escarpment in Ontario, Canada, offering a diverse range of natural landscapes and stunning scenery. The entire trail is marked with white blazes, which are rectangles of white paint usually about 15 cm high and 5 cm wide on trees, fence posts, and rocks. These blazes keep hikers on track and keep us from straying off course.

These blazes are my guideposts. They tell me where to start and the right direction to travel in every time I return to the trail. This same principle applies to your weight-releasing journey—your journey will need a clear path to help you get to your goal.

People often use the phrase "I want to lose weight", believing that this declaration is enough to begin the process. However, deep down they lack clarity about their true desires and the reasons behind them. Just as knowing my starting point and destination along the Bruce Trail is essential for a successful hike, being crystal clear about your health and weight goals is the foundational step to kickstart your journey.

Clarity is the bedrock upon which breakthroughs are built.

What about you? What's your goal?

Over the years of working with people, I've noticed that many often lack the clarity they need regarding what they truly desire in their health. They may have fleeting glimpses or vague ideas, but more often than not these are built on preconceived notions of what an idealized outcome should be. Or, conversely, they never gave it much thought. What's needed to get you started is a clarity that defines your heart's desire, the one that drives you, motivates you, and guides you on this transformative journey. So let's uncover that clarity together and set you on a path to lasting breakthroughs.

Let's go back to my Bruce Trail adventure. On the surface, my goal appeared to be achieving the personal feat of hiking 900 kilometers. But deep down, what I'm truly seeking is a profound sense of accomplishment. I yearn for those moments of peace and solitude when I can connect with God and experience the breathtaking beauty of His creation in all its splendor. It's also an opportunity to live out one of my core values: the thrill of a challenge. As I navigate the twists and turns of the trail I'm embracing the essence of challenge, a value that stirs my soul and reminds me of my innate strength.

In the same way, your weight-releasing journey may seem like a quest for a specific dress size or number on the scale. For you, it may be about the transformation in your spirit, soul and body, and the deep sense of well-being that accompanies each step of your progress. What you truly desire is that wonderful feeling you believe awaits you as you become healthier, right? The truth always lies below the surface, and that's what you're about to discover.

I get it. Right now, you may find it hard to grasp this reality. It seems like an overwhelming task, like you lack what it takes. But today you're taking the first bold and courageous step by gaining clarity about what you genuinely want. Let's turn to God's Word to learn how to achieve this clarity. I've made the process of getting clear super simple by providing you with the very same template we use to help our clients achieve incredible results. Go to breakthroughmethodbonus.com. Simply plug in your own words and start your journey towards lasting transformation.

Write the Vision

> *"Write the vision; make it plain on tablets, so he may run who reads it. For still the vision awaits its appointed time; it hastens to the end—it will not lie. If it seems slow, wait for it; it will surely come; it will not delay." (Hab. 2:2-3 ESV)*

The Book of Habakkuk in the Bible contains a conversation between the prophet Habakkuk and God. In this dialogue, Habakkuk questions God about the apparent injustice and suffering in the world. He is troubled by the wickedness and violence he sees, and seeks answers from God.

In response, God provides a vision to Habakkuk and instructs him to write it down clearly on tablets. The vision pertains to God's plan for justice and the ultimate outcome of the wicked. This passage emphasizes the importance of having a clear vision, committing it to writing and ultimately trusting in God's divine plan, even in times of uncertainty and turmoil. The passage serves as a powerful reminder of the significance of clarity and commitment to your vision.

Habakkuk 2:2 also suggests that a clear vision not only inspires but also propels us into action. The verse mentions, "so he may run who reads it." This implies that when you translate your desires into a well-defined vision, you set the stage for action. You create a compelling narrative that motivates you to take consistent steps towards your goals. It's as if your written vision becomes a catalyst, driving you forward with purpose and determination.

When you commit your goals, desires, and aspirations to writing, you take things to another level. It's more than just putting pen to paper; it's a declaration to yourself that you are serious about your intentions. This simple act of writing down your objectives has a deep impact on your mindset. It signals to your subconscious mind that you are committed, igniting a powerful shift in your mental landscape. This process transforms your hopes and wishes into a concrete vision, something tangible and real. It serves as a roadmap guiding you towards your desired destination.

Now, you may have written down your goals in the past. This is different. Here I'm not just talking about a goal but rather vision. There's a difference.

Your vision is a supernatural revelation from God. It's the culmination of divine guidance, whispers of inspiration, and a sense of purpose that has been with you for as long as you can remember.

God has been speaking to your heart, leading you, and gently directing you towards this vision. It's as though He has been planting seeds of purpose deep within your soul, nurturing them over time until they've grown into a clear, compelling vision.

1. Your vision transcends.

This vision, however, is not limited to a specific aspect of your life; it transcends your health and weight. It encompasses your entire being—body, soul, and spirit. It recognizes that you are a complex and interconnected creation of God, and your vision must reflect that holistic nature.

As you begin crafting your vision, understand that it won't solely revolve around health or weight. It will be a comprehensive, all-encompassing vision that touches every facet of your existence. This vision is God's way of aligning your purpose, desires, and destiny with His divine plan for your life.

So when you sit down to create your vision at the end of this chapter, know that it will be a beautifully intricate tapestry that weaves together the threads of your health, well-being, faith, relationships, and every other aspect of your existence. It's a vision that reflects God's multifaceted design for your life and His desire to see you thrive in every dimension of your being.

2. Your vision is given by God.

God created each of us with a unique purpose, and you will come to discover that your health is intricately tied to fulfilling that purpose.

In our human nature, we sometimes create lofty dreams and set unrealistic goals that often lead to disappointment. We allow our egos to take charge, making decisions that ultimately leave us feeling unfulfilled. We might also let our fears take the wheel, driving our passions and desires in a way that leaves us feeling battered and broken. This pattern can be discouraging and disheartening.

But there's a better way—a way that leads to lasting fulfillment and meaningful progress. When we seek God's guidance and align our vision with His divine plan, we experience a transformational shift. Instead of spinning our wheels in temporary pursuits, we'll be firmly rooted in His purpose for our lives.

As you devote time to connect with God and seek His wisdom, He will reveal to you a breathtaking vision of how you were meticulously designed to live. This vision encompasses not only your physical health but your entire being—mind, body, and spirit. It's a vision that goes beyond the superficial and taps into the depths of your true identity.

3. Your vision is the convergence of hindsight, insight and foresight.

It's a culmination of your past experiences, your present understanding, and your future aspirations.

It's perfectly normal to have reservations about painting a new vision for your life, especially if you've faced disappointments and setbacks in the past. The fear of wanting something and not being able to achieve it can be overwhelmingly painful, and as a result you may have buried your dreams deep within.

But here's the beautiful truth: Your vision isn't just about dreaming for the sake of it. It serves a deeper purpose. It provides you with invaluable insight into your past hurts and disappointments. It allows you to reflect on your journey, understand the lessons learned from your experiences, and identify areas where you may have stumbled or faced challenges.

This process of reflection isn't meant to dwell on the pain of the past but to glean wisdom from it. It's about acknowledging what didn't work, what caused pain, and what hindered your progress. Armed with this understanding, you can craft a new vision—a vision inspired by God Himself.

God's vision for your life is one of healing, growth, and abundance. It's a vision that transcends the limitations of past disappointments and leads you toward a future filled with His grace and purpose. So, as we dive into this transformative journey, I encourage you to cast aside the fear of dreaming again. Instead, embrace the opportunity to create a vision that not only honors your past but also illuminates your path forward—a path guided by God's loving hand.

4. Your vision serves as a powerful bridge.

A bridge that spans the gap between your present circumstances and the future reality you desire.

I understand that, right now, the distance between where you are right now and where you want to be may seem vast. It can appear as though you have an overwhelming journey ahead of you. But I want to assure you of something crucial: God is well aware of this gap, and He has a deep understanding of your potential.

You see, from the very beginning, God created you in His own image (Gen 1:27)—a reflection of His divine qualities and capabilities. You were designed to embody His love, His strength, and His purpose. However, along the twists and turns of life, you may have lost sight of this divine alignment. You may have drifted away from the person God intended you to be.

But here's the remarkable part: As you take hold of your vision for your health, something transformative happens. You begin to look beyond your current circumstances, beyond the challenges and limitations that surround you. You start to believe, truly believe, that you can become all that God says you are.

Your vision becomes a compass that guides you back to your true self—the self that God created with intention and love. Like the blazes on the tree, it will move you forward step by step, inspiring you to reclaim the divine alignment that has always been within you. So embrace your vision for your health with faith and confidence, for it is the key to bridging the gap and becoming the person God destined you to be.

5. Your vision extends far beyond your current circumstances.

I'm sure you've experienced the all-too-familiar pattern of setting your health or weight-release plan into motion, only to see it slowly fade away over time. It's a common experience because, more often than not, these plans are built upon our limited human understanding, unable to encompass the grandeur of God's master plan.

Let me be clear: When we rely solely on our own faculties, our capacity to dream and envision is confined by our human limitations. Our imaginations are bound by the walls of our fears and the constraints of our limiting beliefs. We tend to create plans that align with our current reality, plans that feel safe and attainable.

But here's where it gets truly exciting: When you invite the Holy Spirit into your vision, something remarkable occurs. The Holy Spirit serves as a boundless wellspring of inspiration, empowering you to dream beyond the boundaries of your imagination. It allows you to envision a reality that transcends your current circumstances—a reality that aligns with God's divine plan for your life.

You see, the limitations of your imagination often hold you back from planning for the incredible future that God has in store for you (Jeremiah 29:11).

So be sure to invite the Holy Spirit to guide you as you start writing AND living out the vision you will create for your health. Allow Him to expand your imagination, to help you dream bigger than you ever thought possible. Your vision should be a reflection of God's limitless power and unwavering love for you. It's a vision that transcends your current circumstances, paving the way for God's extraordinary plan to manifest in your life.

6. Your vision is uniquely yours.

I want you to understand that your vision, the one you're about to create, is unlike anyone else's. It's not a cookie-cutter plan or a replica of someone else's journey. It's not based on what you saw on Facebook or read in an Instagram post. Instead, it's a deeply personal and divine revelation—a culmination of the way God has been speaking to you throughout your life.

Your vision takes into account every facet of your being—your values, your personality, your unique gifts, your passions, and your desires. It's a reflection of your true self, aligned with God's purpose for your life. This means your vision cannot be copied or imitated from someone else's. You might be tempted to emulate someone else's path, and it might even seem to work for a while. But sooner or later you'll find yourself returning to your authentic self.

Why is this so important to understand? Because God will never call you to pursue something that He knows you're incapable of achieving. He has designed your vision to perfectly match who you are and what you're capable of.

This unique vision is your guide, your road-map to becoming the best version of yourself.

So embrace the fact that it is uniquely yours! Embrace your individuality, your strengths, and even your limitations. Your vision is tailor-made for you, and it's a beautiful reflection of God's intricate design for your life. Trust that it will lead you exactly where you need to go.

7. Your vision impacts generations to come.

As you get clearer on your vision, I encourage you to think beyond yourself and your immediate circumstances. Consider the people within your circle of influence—the ones who look up to you, especially your children and even your children's children. It's at this point that you'll truly grasp the significance of having a vision.

You may have encountered this principle in a negative light, perhaps by inheriting certain health challenges like high blood pressure or diabetes from your parents. But here's the remarkable opportunity: you have the power to break that cycle. You can choose to model and pass on a new level of health to the next generation.

Imagine being the one to initiate a positive shift in your family's health legacy. Picture your children and grandchildren inheriting a legacy of wellness, purpose, and vitality instead of the history of illnesses that may have plagued your family for generations. Your decision to craft a new vision for your health and follow through with it can be the pivotal moment when a new legacy begins.

Let me respectfully say that it isn't just about you—it's about the lasting impact your vision will have on those who come after you. You have the ability to create a new narrative, one filled with health, faith, and inspiration. So as you write your vision, remember that you're not only shaping your own future but also influencing the generations to come. You are indeed creating a legacy of health and wholeness.

8 . Your vision will take you out of your comfort zone.

Now, let's talk about an important aspect of creating your vision—it will challenge you to step out of your comfort zone. Too often people delay, downsize, or even completely derail their dreams simply because they're afraid to dream boldly. They play it small and safe, underestimating the immense cost of a life not fully lived.

It's a harsh reality that many individuals will quietly journey through life without ever realizing the fullness of God's best for them. Why does this happen? Well, because stepping out of our comfort zone is inherently risky. Questions like "What if it doesn't work?" or "What if I fail?" often plague our minds.

Let's be honest: if fulfilling our God-given vision was easy, we'd all be living our best lives effortlessly. The fitness industry wouldn't be a billion-dollar business, and our medical bills would be significantly lower. The truth is, success in any endeavor requires hard work, discipline, consistency, and un-wavering determination.

We owe it to ourselves to stay the course and live the healthy life we were de-signed for. Yet stepping out of your comfort zone is a challenge. It demands extra effort and, if we're honest with ourselves, we're often unprepared to put in that level of work. Moreover, stepping out of your comfort zone neces-sitates relinquishing control of your current situation and trusting God to show you His way.

I won't sugarcoat it—it's impossible to fully embrace the gift of good health and remain entirely comfortable. Getting healthier requires discipline, sac-rifice, and a whole lot of sweat equity. However, I can promise you this: it's worth it. *You* are worth it.

9. Your vision is grounded in reality.

It's crucial to distinguish your vision from whimsical wishes, idle wanting, or mere hope that life was different. You may have ventured down those paths before, and you've likely discovered that they lead to feelings of guilt and frustration. Wishing without purpose and hoping without a plan can become a cycle of unfulfilled desires.

Your vision, on the other hand, is firmly grounded in reality. It's not about escaping your current circumstances but transforming them. It's about ac-knowledging where you are now and taking purposeful steps to reach where you want to be. Your vision is a road-map to a better, healthier, and more fulfilling life.

By embracing the reality of your current situation with grace and compassion, you set the stage for meaningful change. You can't build a solid bridge to your future if you're not standing firmly on the ground of your present.

10 . Your vision must be based on trusting God's Word.

Now let's conclude with an essential aspect of crafting your vision—it must be rooted in your unwavering trust in God's Word. This might seem obvious, but it's worth emphasizing. Without placing your trust in God, you're essentially jotting down a list of hopeful wants, wishes, and desires that are unlikely to come to fruition. You might experience fleeting success, but it rarely endures.

In the Book of Habakkuk, God conveyed to the prophet Habakkuk that the vision He provided would indeed come to pass, and Habakkuk wholeheartedly believed God's word. This principle is encapsulated in the phrase, "the righteous will live by faith" (Habakkuk 2:4). Faith is, at its core, about what you truly believe.

In the context of your health and weight-release journey, your vision must be underpinned by your unwavering faith in God's promises. It's not just about wishful thinking. It's about firmly trusting that God will guide you, empower you, and lead you to your envisioned destination. By anchoring your vision in God's Word, you fortify it with the strength and resilience to withstand the trials and challenges that may arise on your journey. Your faith will be the driving force behind your vision's transformation from a mere idea to a tangible reality.

Continuing on, it may seem like I've emphasized this point extensively, but having a vision for your health is truly that crucial. It forms the cornerstone of your journey. To help you streamline the process of crafting your vision, we'll take a practical approach. Now, with that solid foundation, let's begin to craft your vision for your health.

Writing Your Vision

To write your vision, you're going to create a snapshot of one day in your life when you've living at your healthy weight. Picture it in vivid detail. What do you want to feel and experience each day? How does that day unfold from the moment you wake up?

As you close your eyes and envision this day, immerse yourself in the experience. What are you doing? Who are you with? Feel the emotions that bubble up as you move through this day. Is it a day filled with energy, vitality, and joy? Visualize the activities, the food choices, and the interactions that make up this ideal day.

By breaking it down into a single day, you make your vision more tangible and achievable. It's a practical exercise that brings your aspirations into focus. This day serves as a compass, guiding you towards your desired destination.

Remember, this is your vision; uniquely yours. It doesn't need to conform to anyone else's expectations or ideals. It's a reflection of your desires, your values, and your dreams for a healthier and happier you. So as you embark on this journey of vision crafting, immerse yourself in that future day and let it be a source of inspiration and motivation.

Suggestions for Writing Your Vision

1. Focus on how you want to feel.

First and foremost, focus on how you want to feel. Your health journey is about so much more than just shedding pounds; it's about gaining a life filled with vitality, confidence, freedom, joy, longevity, and self-love. These are the experiences that truly matter and will sustain your motivation.

Imagine waking up each morning feeling invigorated, confident in your skin, and free from the burdens that excess weight can bring. Envision a life where joy radiates from within, where you're not just living but thriving. Picture yourself enjoying a long, fulfilling life, cherishing each moment and extending your journey's blessings to future generations.

As you write your vision, let these feelings guide your words. Describe the emotions, sensations, and fulfillment you'll experience on this journey. Your vision will be a testament to your incredible transformation.

By focusing on how you want to feel, your vision becomes a powerful motivator, a source of inspiration that will keep you aligned with your goals and committed to the path ahead.

2. Engage as many of your senses as possible

When writing out your vision for your health, make the process as vivid and sensory-rich as possible. Engaging multiple senses in your vision can make it more tangible and emotionally resonant, helping you stay committed to your goals. Here's how you can do it:

Visualize the Scenery. Imagine the surroundings of your healthier life. Describe the vibrant colors of the fruits and vegetables on your plate, the serene view from your morning yoga spot, or the lush greenery on your jogging route. Visual details can make your vision more captivating.

Taste and Smell. Incorporate vivid descriptions of taste and smell into your vision. Imagine savoring a delicious, nourishing meal. Describe the aroma of your favorite nutritious dishes, the scent of herbs and spices, or the freshness of your morning smoothie. These sensory experiences can make your vision mouthwatering and enjoyable.

Physical Sensations. Consider how it feels to be in a healthier body. Describe the sensation of your muscles working during a workout, the refreshing feeling of water after a good sweat, or the warmth of a post-exercise shower.

Auditory Elements. Don't forget to include sounds in your vision. Imagine the rhythm of your heartbeat during exercise, the soothing music playing in your earphones while you're walking, the birds chirping, the sounds of the waves as you walk on the beach, or the laughter and conversations with friends during a nutritious meal. Auditory cues can bring your vision to life.

Emotions and Achievements. Describe the emotions you'll experience in your day—the pride, the joy, the sense of accomplishment. Paint a picture of the moments when you reach milestones like crossing a finish line, hitting a personal best, or simply feeling at peace with your body.

By engaging as many senses as possible, your vision for a healthier life becomes a multi-dimensional, sensory-rich experience. This can help make your goals more tangible, relatable, and motivating. It brings your vision to life in a way that inspires and fuels your commitment to a healthier you.

3. State it in the present.

Writing in the present tense creates a powerful and positive affirmation of your intentions. It reinforces the idea that your vision is not a distant future, but something you are actively and confidently working towards in the present moment. "I wake up in the morning." "I go for a walk". Do not use statements like "I will", "I would be", "I hope", "I want to", or "I will no longer be lazy."

4. State everything in the positive tense.

Writing your health goals in the positive tense is crucial because it shifts your focus from what you want to avoid to what you want to achieve, providing clear direction and empowering you to take control of your journey. Positive statements not only reinforce a sense of urgency and accomplishment but also cultivate a more optimistic and motivated mindset. They serve as daily affirmations, counteracting negative self-talk and limiting beliefs. By framing your goals positively you maintain a forward-looking perspective, highlighting the possibilities and opportunities for growth in your health journey.

Instead of saying "I will be pain-free", say, "My body moves with ease" or "I feel energized."

Instead of saying, "I will no longer obsess about my weight," say, "I focus on what really matters", or "I enjoy the freedom of being at a healthy weight."

Instead of saying, "I will be less self-conscious", say "I love the confidence I experience knowing that the Lord is my strength."

5. Don't be afraid to dream.

I've heard so many women say that they're afraid to see God because they're afraid that He's going to tell them to do something that they don't want to do.

I encourage you to trust and believe that God is not going to lead you somewhere without preparing you first. He's not going to send you out to a mission field in the jungles of Africa if you pass out at the sight of a bug, and He's not going to tell you to become a vegetarian if you live on a farm, raise livestock for a living, and love all things meat. So before God can entrust you with a vision, you have to get clear on where you are right now and where God is leading you—which is different from where you think God is leading you or where you want to go.

6. Don't make it a list of what you will and will not do. Focus on the things that bring you joy.

It's important not to turn your vision into a list of "dos and don'ts" and instead focus on what brings you joy for several compelling reasons. When your vision reads like a to-do list, it can feel restrictive and uninspiring, potentially leading to a sense of obligation rather than enthusiasm.

In contrast, emphasizing joyful activities and experiences in your vision ignites your passion and enthusiasm for your health journey. This approach makes your vision more exciting, motivating, and sustainable as you look forward to engaging in activities that bring happiness and fulfillment. Additionally, when your vision centers on joy it aligns with the belief that God's best for you includes a life filled with positivity, contentment and delight, further reinforcing your faith and commitment to your health goals.

7. Incorporate all aspects of your life.

Although it is a health vision your vision incorporates all aspects of your life, so be sure to include them all. Select a day that will incorporate as many different aspects of your life as possible. It could be a day on vacation, on the weekend, time with your family or friends, or operating in your giftings—maybe you're speaking to thousands of women, or operating your business, caring for your children, signing books, or serving in the mission field. Include the things that God has put on your heart to do. As you think about your future, what activities are you doing with your family or your loved ones? How are they benefiting from your renewed vitality? Be sure to include them in your vision.

Now it's time to put pen to paper and start writing. This is your first step, so please don't skip it. You can visit breakthroughmethodbonus.com to look at some of our sample visions that our members created. Use it to help you spark some ideas of your own.

Principle 1 Summary

Reflect on these key points:

- **Clarity is essential.** Your health journey begins with a clear understanding of what you truly desire, beyond surface-level weight loss goals.

- **Embrace your deeper desires.** Look beyond shedding pounds to seek freedom, peace, confidence, and joy in your health journey.

- **Write your vision.** Commit your health goals to writing, ensuring they reflect your deepest desires, engage your senses, and encompass all aspects of your life.

Principle #2: Maximize Your Energy

Honor Your Core Four

Now that you've set your course for your desired destination, let's explore a radically different approach to achieving it. In the past, on your weight loss journey, you likely followed the conventional path of calorie restriction and increased exercise, which, while admirable, often proves to be unsustainable in the long run, as you may have personally experienced. What's even more concerning is that calorie reduction or excessive exercise can actually slow down your metabolism and trigger heightened appetite. This happens because your body maintains a natural set point, and significant fluctuations can disrupt its delicate balance.

As I reminisce about some of those hikes along the Bruce Trail, I have fond memories of some invigorating and uplifting adventures. These were the ones where I packed enough water and snacks, had a restful night's sleep, wore the right clothing and wool socks that didn't chafe my feet, and listened to my body by taking breaks when I needed them. I also focused on the beautiful sights and sounds instead of complaining about the less desirable aspect like bugs and achy feet. When all these factors were in place, my energy was optimized and I moved steadily along the paths—blazing the trails. On the other hand, there were hikes that couldn't be over fast enough. My energy was low and every step felt like I was carrying a 200-pound sack on my back. As I think back, these are the ones where I was super-exhausted from staying up too late the night before, or in some way I was not prepared for the journey at hand. The difference was usually in one of these four areas which are affectionately known in Weight Loss, God's Way as "The Core Four".

These "Core Four" will also be foundations in your health and weight releasing journey. They are four fundamental pillars just like the cornerstone of a strong and stable foundation that will support your journey toward a healthier and more vibrant you.

Effective Stress Management. Stress is an ever-present force in our lives, and how we manage it impacts our overall health. Mastering stress isn't just about finding moments of calm; it's about aligning your spirit, soul, and body. When you effectively manage stress you help balance those hunger hormones once more, ensuring that you're in sync with your divine purpose and the goals you've set for yourself.

Healthy Eating. Think of your body as a finely tuned machine created by the Master Himself. To function at its best, it needs the right fuel. Healthy eating isn't solely about shedding pounds; it's about nurturing your body with nutrient-rich foods, consumed at the right times and in appropriate portions. By nourishing your body in this way, you're not only promoting natural weight release but also unlocking boundless energy and assisting your body in returning to its natural, God-given state.

Physical Activity. The human body is designed for movement. Regular physical activity isn't just about managing weight; it's about optimizing every system within you. Exercise keeps your muscles strong, your heart healthy, and your mind sharp. It's a vital component of your journey toward overall well-being and an essential part of the Core Four.

Adequate Sleep. Quality sleep is a secret weapon on your weight-releasing journey. While you rest your body is hard at work, balancing hunger hormones, repairing and rejuvenating cells, and supercharging your energy levels. It's during deep, restful sleep that your body has the chance to recalibrate, setting the stage for a successful and healthy weight release.

Throughout this book, I'll consistently emphasize that the Core Four principles aren't merely a temporary fix but a way of life. They hold the key to unlocking your energy potential, enabling you to optimize your performance and overall health. You will discover how to seamlessly incorporate these principles into your daily routine, leading to both the shedding of excess weight and a transformation in how you feel, look, and live.

There's a poignant Biblical story that highlights the critical importance of performance optimization and energy maximization. While it's a cautionary tale, we can draw valuable lessons from it.

The tale centers around David, a remarkable figure who faced numerous battles throughout his life, including battles with the Moabites, Geshurites, Gezrites, and, of course, the dreaded "cellulites". I couldn't resist adding the last one! Who knows, even Biblical heroes might have had their battles with those stubborn little foes, too!

Anyhow, back to the story.

For years, King Saul relentlessly pursued David, forcing him to flee for his life with six hundred men and their families into Philistine territory. Here, Achish, the Philistine king of Gath, granted David's request for the town of Ziklag.

David ruled Ziklag for sixteen months, using it as a strategic base for military campaigns against the Amalekites. However, a turning point occurred when the Amalekites raided Ziklag, reducing it to ashes and capturing women and children.

> *"Then David returned to the brook Besor and met up with the 200 men who had been left behind because they were too exhausted to go with him." (1 Samuel 30:21 NLT)*

In a daring rescue mission David and his men pursued the raiders, ultimately recovering everything that had been taken. However, it's notable that 200 of his men remained at the Brook Besor because, as the scripture tells us, they were 'too exhausted to continue'! Can you fathom the situation? Your loved ones and possessions have been captured, yet you're too fatigued to fight for what's rightfully yours? This moment at the Brook Besor serves as a stark reminder of the critical role energy plays in our ability to pursue our goals and overcome challenges. It's a powerful example of how energy management can make the difference between success and stagnation on your journey to better health and fulfilling your God-given purpose.

The Brook Besor serves as an analogy for your own journey, a test of your energy management. It represents those critical moments on your path when your strength is put to the ultimate test. It's the point where you must decide whether you have the vigor to advance and seize all that God has in store for you or recognize that you need a transformation in your energy management.

Your assignment is too significant to be hindered by lack of energy. That's why you're here. You're going to develop a lifestyle that empowers you to carry on and fulfill your God-given purpose. Just as David and his men faced their defining moment at the Brook Besor, you too must embrace the challenge, ensuring you have the vitality to press on and embrace all that God has ordained for your journey.

That's precisely why this fresh outlook is so significant. Your journey will now prioritize energy management, self-care, stewardship, and empowerment instead of weight loss. You'll learn how to embrace your role as the devoted custodian of your body, recognizing it as God's sacred temple, deserving of the highest degree of care and nourishment. Your primary objective will be to find ways to maximize your daily energy levels in these four areas of your life. This approach will enable you to address the deeper issues that have been driving your behavior instead of merely managing the symptoms which for you has manifested as excess weight.

But here's the great news: You're not alone in this journey. As you surrender this journey to God, He will give you everything you need to be successful. As you shift your focus towards vitality and energy, you'll find a renewed sense of purpose and a healthier, more empowered version of yourself emerging. It's about stepping into your God-given potential, fueled by the energy and strength that come from caring for your God-given temple. So let's explore this path together, eager to uncover the true source of lasting change—maximizing your energy, and in turn allowing your body to find its right size and optimal health.

A Powerful Question You Must Ask Yourself: Does this Maximize My Energy?

I want to give you a simple but powerful self-coaching tip to carry forward in your journey. For simplicity and clarity, we'll call it the Energy Evaluator throughout the rest of this book. Ask yourself, *'Does this maximize my energy?'* This simple question, rooted in the Core Four principles, will guide you in making choices that prioritize energy management over other factors like cravings, calories, convenience, or complacency.

When it comes to making food choices, ask yourself, **"Does this maximize my energy?"** This question shifts the focus from indulgence to nourishing your body with nutrient-rich foods.

Ask yourself, "Does this maximize my energy?" when planning your workouts. This question guides you to choose activities that invigorate you rather than drain you. Opt for exercises that leave you feeling empowered and recharged, as opposed to ones that exhaust you. This might range from stressing to sweating.

When coping with life's challenges, ask yourself, "Does this choice I'm about to make maximize my energy?" This query helps you find ways to reduce stress and maintain a healthy emotional balance. Asking yourself this question is also a good reminder for you to check in with yourself and make sure that you've invited God into your challenging situations and circumstances. Nothing robs your energy more than striving and struggling trying to fix yourself and your stressful circumstances.

Lastly, as you make choices around creating a positive sleep environment, ask yourself, "Does this maximize my energy?" This will help you to make informed decisions about what you should and should not do, such as drink that cup of coffee at 8:00 pm or start watching that Netflix series.

In the coming chapters, we'll spend time breaking down all of these pillars in detail.

Health as Stewardship

If the Core Four represents 'what' you will do to help you move towards optimal health, your motivation will determine your 'why'. Motivation is the driving force behind your actions. It's the deep, meaningful reasons that inspire you to make healthier choices, prioritize your well-being, and stay dedicated to your journey. Understanding your motivation is key, as it will be your steadfast companion on your journey.

What motivates you now? Or maybe that's your challenge, you lack motivation. What if your motivation to lose weight was grounded in God? What if the focus were on effective stewardship of your temple?

Understand, unequivocally, that your weight holds significance in the eyes of God, but maybe not in the ways that you might think. God does not care how much you weigh, BUT it goes much deeper than that.

The Bible is not silent on the topic. Here are some scriptures that talk about behaviors that lead to excess weight:

> *Proverbs 23:20 (KJV): "Be not among drunkards or among gluttonous eaters of meat."*
>
> *Proverbs 28:7 (KJV): "A companion of gluttons shames his father."*
>
> *Philippians 3:19 (KJV): "Their end is destruction, their god is their belly, and thy glory is their shame, with minds set on earthly things."*
>
> *Proverbs 23:2 (KJV): "And put a knife to thy throat, if thou be a man given to appetite [controlled by appetite]."*

I share these scriptures not to make you feel bad, but it's strictly for those who sometimes don't believe God cares about this area of our lives.

Sometimes, you may find yourself doubting whether God truly cares about this particular aspect of your life. It's possible that, without realizing it, you've used Scripture to downplay the importance of prioritizing a healthy lifestyle. This self-imposed limitation is unfortunate because it's precisely when you are healthy, energized, confident, and feeling your best that the light of Christ radiates even more brilliantly for others to witness.

It's crucial to understand that investing in your well-being is neither vain nor fruitless. In fact, making your physical health a priority will have implications for your overall life. When you neglect your health, you risk being confronted by sickness and disease, which demand far more of your time and energy in the long run. These health challenges can also impose limitations on your ability to fulfill your kingdom assignment.

By recognizing the significance of tending to your physical well-being, you not only honor the body that God has entrusted you with but also position yourself to be a more effective instrument of His love, grace, and purpose in the world. In caring for your health you are better equipped to serve others, shine His light, and fulfill the calling He has placed upon your life.

There are two scriptures that can lead us into believing that we should not focus on our physical bodies:

> *"For the Lord sees not as man sees: man looks on the outward appearance, but the Lord looks on the heart" (1 Samuel 16:7 ESV),*

and

> *"For physical training is of some value, but godliness has value for all things, holding promise for both the present life and the life to come" (1 Tim 4:8 (NIV)).*

It's true that both of these scriptures place a higher value on your inner man, your heart, and your soul. Know that God also cares about your 'outer man', which is how the Bible refers to your body. The second verse says that physical training has value. It does not say what some of us think it says, that physical training is unimportant and worthless.

Based on these two scriptures, you can be led to think that God does not care if you're unhealthy, but if you dig deeper you can see that this is not the case.

Let's look at some of the things the Bible tells us that God cares about in relation to your health:

Your health matters to God because **God cares about whatever keeps you from fulfilling your purpose and destiny**. Ephesians 2:10 tells us that "*We are His workmanship, created in Christ Jesus for good works, which God prepared beforehand that we should walk in them*" (ESV). First, we are His workmanship. How amazing is that?

He created you for good works, but you may feel so bound by your weight. You may be physically and emotionally unable to walk in your anointing because your weight is a hindrance. Or it may be the sense of shame that keeps you from fully embracing your God-given calling. Be encouraged by the thought that God has prepared good works for you to do. Use this knowledge for deeper motivation and inspiration to get healthier. What has God called you to do? Keep that in front of you and use it as a driving force to live your best and healthiest life in service of your anointing.

Your health matters to God because **God cares about what you care about.** One of my favorite scriptures is found in 1 Peter 5:7: "Cast all your anxiety on Him, because He cares for you." It reminds me that God cares about everything I care about; everything that worries me and causes me anxiety. Being overweight can be all-consuming. It occupies space and time that God wants. If you're overweight and it's causing you stress and anxiety, then know that God cares about this also. He does not want you stressed or anxious, and wants you to get the help you need so you are at peace.

Your health matters to God because **your body belongs to Him.**

We live in a culture that tells you that your body is yours to do with whatever you please, as long as you're not hurting anyone, but God's Word tells you differently. From the beginning to the end of the Bible, Scripture tells you that God owns everything, including your body. Everything you do to and with your body concerns God because He created your body, and loaned it to you to live in while you are here on Earth.

> *"Do you not know that your bodies are temples of the Holy Spirit, who is in you, whom you have received from God? You are not your own; you were bought at a price. Therefore honor God with your bodies." (1 Cor 6:19-20 NIV)*

It's important to reflect on this with compassion. Since your body doesn't belong solely to you, you're not entirely free to treat it without consideration. You hold a responsibility to care for it. When you begin to view your body as something you are entrusted to steward on behalf of God, it can inspire a pause and a shift in your perspective.

Your weight holds significance to God because how you nurture and manage your body during your earthly existence has a lasting impact on eternity.

> *"So we make it our goal to please him, whether we are at home in the body or away from it" (2 Corinthians 5:9 NIV).*

When you transition from solely considering your immediate needs to contemplating life in the context of eternity, a great shift occurs within your values and priorities.

Consider this: If this earthly life were all there was, you might feel inclined to indulge in every desire, especially when it comes to food, with the belief that your actions have no long-term repercussions. However, we must remember that life extends beyond the here and now. Every choice you make, every action you take while on this Earth, holds the potential for lasting impact in eternity

Let this realization serve as a guiding light, illuminating the importance of nurturing your tripartite being—your spirit, soul, and body. It's an acknowledgment that the choices you make today, including how you care for your body, can resonate through the ages, influencing not just your own journey but also leaving a mark in the grand design of eternity.

In his book *The Purpose Driven Life*, Rick Warren says: "Life on earth is just a dress rehearsal for the real production. Earth is the staging area, the pre-school, the tryout for your life in eternity. We will only be motivated to make good choices each day when we're convinced that everything we do here on earth, including taking care of your temple matters to God. If we don't believe it then why should you be a steward of your body? Why don't we just eat whatever we want and do whatever we please? God will judge you on what you did with what he gave you here on Earth. I heard someone say to "live each day as if Jesus is coming back at any moment and plan your life like He isn't coming back for 100 years."

> *"The world and its desires pass away, but whoever does the will of God lives forever." (1 John 2:17 NIV)*

Believe that your body is God's temple, and you begin to see just how important it is to take care of it. You'll see that your reasons and motivation to be healthy go far deeper than just the number on the scale.

Your health matters to God because **God cares about your total health, not just the spiritual aspects.** In 1 Thes. 5:23, the Apostle Paul divides human nature into three parts—spirit, soul, and body, and prays to God on behalf of the converts. *"May God himself, the God of peace, sanctify you through and through. May your whole spirit, soul and body be kept blameless at the coming of our Lord Jesus Christ."* Let us also pray to God that all aspects of our human nature be sanctified and strengthened.

God wants you to glorify Him in your body. It's our physical bodies that cause us much trouble. Imagine if you did not have physical bodies. Imagine no insecurity issues, jealousy issues, gluttony issues, lust issues, right? Yet your Father saw fit to give you a physical body that would glorify Him. Your responsibility (reasonable service) is to keep it holy by taking care of it. In Romans 12:1, Paul addresses the crowd by stating: *"I beseech you therefore, brethren, by the mercies of God, that ye present your bodies a living sacrifice, holy, acceptable unto God, which is your reasonable service"* (NKJV).

God most certainly cares about your health. Not in a 'you should be a size 8, not 18' sort of way, or in a way that is overly concerned about whether you're the right proportions. His care and love for you extend far beyond anything that you can comprehend.

He cares because He knows that being healthy will have an impact on generations to come (1 Kings 15:3).

He cares because your outer body is a physical manifestation of what's going on inside your mind and spirit. He wants to free you of the bondage and challenges that come with it. That's what the power of His Word can do (Hebrews 4:12).

He cares because taking care of your health (like our finances, relationships, family, and careers) are seeds that, when managed well, increase your capacity for impact and prepare you for greater things to come (Luke 16:10).

Now with these new truths in mind, I pray that you will begin to pursue your health with a new sense of urgency and understanding. Shift your perspective; see the bigger picture. Your entire life fits into a much larger picture, and this stronghold is so consuming it's limiting your vision and ability to see beyond this immediate need.

When you come to embrace the truth that extends beyond mere weight loss—realizing that God's purpose is to mold your character and fortify your inner self—something transformative happens. You cease to abandon your journey every time a setback emerges on your path. Instead, you discover that your pursuit of weight release becomes a vessel for nurturing the fruits of the Spirit within you.

Consider these divine qualities: love, not just for others but also for yourself; peace, which extends to your relationship with both yourself and your body; patience, graciously granted to the process; kindness, tenderly bestowed upon yourself; faith, not only in your own capabilities but also in God's unwavering desire to assist you; and self-control, gently exercised in your approach to eating (Galatians 5:22).

As these fruits blossom within you, the journey toward weight release is no longer a daunting struggle. Instead, it becomes a journey of stewardship, obedience, spiritual transformation, and lasting self-care.

Empower Your Purpose

I used to read about the Proverbs 31 woman with a mix of jealousy, disdain, guilt, and dread. She was the spiritual Barbie of the Bible, perfect in every way yet unrealistic and unattainable to most. If you're not familiar with the scripture, it paints a vivid picture of a woman who's got it going on. Wife, mother, business woman, home-maker, smart, and sexy. She even finds time to work out! The author is unknown but it's said to be written by King Solomon from the advice given to him by his mother.

Then one day I happened to be reading the chapter again—it was probably yet another Mother's Day message and verse 17 in the Amplified Bible landed for me very differently than it had in the past.

"She girds herself with strength [spiritual, mental, and physical fitness for her God-given task] and makes her arms strong and firm." (Proverbs 31:17 AMPC)

What a revelation the Lord gave me that day! She strengthens herself for her God-given tasks. That's how she was able to accomplish so much. That's what keeps her going. That's her 'why'. She is on assignment, fulfilling her God-given assignment. That's the shift I continue to make in my life, and I'm extending that same invitation for you to join me.

Just as the Proverbs 31 woman dedicates herself to nurturing and enhancing her spiritual, mental, and physical strength, you, too, can adopt a holistic approach to health. Like her, you will also learn that your body, soul, and spirit are interwoven facets of your being, each serving a unique purpose in your God-given journey.

Just as the Proverbs 31 woman prepares herself for her God-given responsibilities, your journey can also be one of preparation and stewardship. By embracing this holistic view of health, you not only honor God's temple but also equip yourself to serve Him more effectively in the God-given tasks and assignments He has designed specifically for you. It's a huge shift that I pray empowers you to approach health not as a superficial pursuit but as a sacred responsibility—one that encompasses the totality of your being, reflecting God's intention for your entire being.

Let this verse also encourage you to shift your perspective and inspire you to gird yourself for your God-given tasks in all areas of your life. By doing so, you can break free from the cycle of yo-yo dieting, chronic stress, and inconsistent habits. Instead, you will prioritize maximizing your energy levels, aligning with your God-given purpose, and pursuing a healthier and more fulfilling life

Indeed, it might be a radical departure from what you've tried in the past, but let's consider it in a different light. You've been struggling to maintain your health goals because they often revolve around your wants (or lack of), needs, and desires. But when you reframe your health goals as an act of stewardship and pursuit of your God-given tasks, you anchor them in a deeper, more meaningful purpose.

Just as a steward diligently cares for and manages valuable possessions entrusted to them, you are called to steward your body. By doing so, you ensure that you have the physical strength, endurance, and vitality needed to fulfill the unique assignments God has planned for your life. And the bonus is that your body will find its naturally healthy size as it moves with purpose and intention every day.

Consider this: When you prioritize your health as an act of stewardship, you're not only investing in yourself but also in your capacity to serve and make a difference in the lives of others. Your health becomes a tool, a vessel through which you can carry out God's work with vigor and dedication.

Principle 2 Summary

Reflect on these key points:

- Prioritize energy management over weight loss by honoring the Core Four. Continually ask yourself, does this maximize my energy?
- Prioritize stewardship over personal wants, needs, and desires.
- Know and believe that God cares about your health.

Principle #3: Calm Your Nervous System

Let Go and Let God

Let Go and Let God

In this chapter, we'll explore the first of the Core Four in detail: stress management. Although all four pillars are important, how we manage our stress is probably the most important of the four pillars because it's the linchpin that holds the other three pillars. While adequate sleep, healthy eating, and physical activity are vital components of a healthy lifestyle, they can all be significantly influenced by stress.

Stress has become a pervasive issue in our modern lives, and when left unchecked it can wreak havoc on our bodies. Stress in and of itself is a natural response designed to help us react to threats and challenges. However, the chronic and unrelenting stress that many people experience today is what poses significant health risks.

Unfortunately and ironically, we don't prioritize stress management because it's a blind spot for so many of us. We've normalized and even glamorize our stress by using terms like "I'm on my grind" and "Burning the midnight oil" but this is not God's best for us. In fact, God gives us a model of work in how He created the Earth and then rested. By the end of this chapter, my hope is that you will learn to live and approach your health from a place of ease and grace.

The Power of Releasing

In your journey toward better health, you may have found yourself in a battle of willpower, constantly resisting the very things you desire. It's a struggle most of us face, and I want you to know that it's not your fault. Our diet culture has seduced us into believing that we need to resist certain foods, resist cravings, resist the discomfort of exercise, and even resist facing the emotional factors that contribute to our struggles. It only makes sense that you should resist temptation, right? Even the Bible teaches us that (James 4:7, 1 Peter 5:9, Eph 4:27). However, nowhere in the Bible does it tell us that we are to resist anything in our own strength. And that's where we've tripped ourselves up. It's God's power in us that gives us the strength to resist temptations.

In fact, Scripture warns against the dangers of change without first filling yourself with God's power. You need to fill yourself with God's power, His guidance, and His strength. It's through a reliance on Him that you find the true strength to resist temptation and make positive changes in your journey to better health.

"When an evil spirit leaves a person, it goes into the desert, seeking rest but finding none. Then it says, 'I will return to the person I came from.' So it returns and finds its former home empty, swept, and in order. Then the spirit finds seven other spirits more evil than itself, and they all enter the person and live there. And so that person is worse off than before." (Matthew 12:43-45) Your own personal experience might have confirmed this principle. You've tried to resist with all your might and you did well for a bit, only to find that the cravings came back even more powerful than before.

Your approach to releasing weight can either work in harmony with your body or, inadvertently, resist the very weight loss you're striving to achieve. As you continue reading, you'll come to understand the relationship between stress and weight and see why your anxiety-producing approach to releasing weight can actually be the very thing that's keeping you stuck. Or, in many cases, worse off than before.

That's why one of our mottoes at Weight Loss, God's Way is: "What you resist persists, and what you release flows with ease." Stressful approaches to losing weight keep you stuck in a never-ending cycle. In this chapter and throughout this book, you will learn how to approach your journey with acceptance, ease, and grace.

There's an oft-repeated parable about how hunters catch monkeys in Africa. The hunters place a jar of peanuts at the base of the tree to lure the monkeys. When a monkey puts its hand in the jar to take out the peanuts, it finds that it is unable to take its fisted hand out of the jar without letting go of the peanuts. It is said that the monkey will remain for hours until it gets caught because it does not want to let go of the peanuts. Though this seems like an illogical action for such intelligent creatures, we too get trapped because we cling so dearly to what we desperately want and are unwilling to release. We forcefully try to control our lives and our circumstances instead of using our intuition, faith, wisdom, and God-given power. Let me show you how this very behavior has been negatively impacting your health and weight.

Impact of Stress on Your Weight

I am committed to helping you break down your old beliefs about health so that you can erect a new Biblical and holistic approach to your health. In order to do that, you should understand how your current mindset about stress may be currently sabotaging you.

Let's look at into the physiological, emotional, and spiritual rationale behind why stress management isn't just a luxury but a crucial component of our journey towards releasing excess weight and embracing a healthier lifestyle.

Physiologically

Cortisol and Fat Storage: Stress triggers the release of cortisol, which is your body's primary stress hormone. Elevated cortisol levels can lead to the storage of visceral fat, particularly around the abdominal region. This type of fat is associated with an increased risk of various health conditions, including cardiovascular diseases and insulin resistance. Managing stress is important for mitigating these adverse effects on body composition and overall health.

Insulin Resistance: Chronic stress contributes to insulin resistance, a condition where cells become less responsive to insulin's effects. This can result in higher blood sugar levels and an increased likelihood of weight gain. When stress management becomes an integral part of your daily routine it can aid in maintaining insulin sensitivity, supporting better blood sugar control and weight management.

Hormonal Imbalance: Stress disrupts hormonal balance, affecting key hormones involved in regulating hunger and fullness. Leptin, the hormone responsible for signaling satiety, can be affected by chronic stress, leading to overeating and a skewed perception of fullness. Additionally, ghrelin, the hormone that stimulates appetite, may become dysregulated, further contributing to unhealthy eating habits. Managing stress can help restore hormonal balance and improve appetite control.

Inflammation and Metabolism: Stress activates the body's inflammatory response, which, when chronic, can interfere with metabolic processes. Inflammatory signals can disrupt the efficient utilization of calories and contribute to weight gain. Stress management strategies, such as relaxation techniques and regular physical activity, play a vital role in reducing chronic inflammation, thereby supporting healthy metabolism.

Muscle Breakdown: Stress can promote the breakdown of muscle tissue and hinder muscle growth. Maintaining lean muscle mass is essential for a healthy metabolism, as muscle tissue burns more calories at rest compared to fat tissue. Chronic stress-induced muscle loss can slow down your weight loss efforts and reduce overall energy expenditure. Incorporating resistance training and stress reduction practices can help preserve and build muscle mass.

Sleep Disruption: Stress often goes hand-in-hand with sleep disturbances, leading to poor sleep quality and insufficient rest. Inadequate sleep resulting from stress can disrupt hormonal regulation, appetite control, and energy levels. These disruptions can negatively impact your weight management efforts. Prioritizing sleep hygiene and stress management techniques can help improve sleep patterns and enhance overall well-being.

Emotionally

Cravings and Emotional Eating: Stress has a direct impact on your cravings and eating patterns. During stressful situations your body tends to crave high-calorie, sugary, and fatty foods, often leading to emotional eating as a coping mechanism. These emotional-eating episodes can sabotage weight-release efforts and result in weight gain over time. Learning to iden-tify and address emotional triggers through stress management can signifi-cantly improve your relationship with food.

Spiritually

The list is long for how stress can impact your relationship with God.

Tests Your Trust: Stressful situations can test your trust in God's plan and timing. The uncertainty and discomfort of these moments may lead you to question whether God is truly present and attentive to your needs. Devel-oping resilience through prayer and meditation can help you navigate these challenging times while strengthening your faith.

Shifts Priorities: Stress may shift your focus from your spiritual journey to immediate problems. The urgency of stressful situations can lead you to prioritize temporary solutions over your long-term spiritual growth.

Struggles with Surrender: Stressful times can challenge your ability to sur-render your worries to God. The desire for control may intensify, making it harder to release your concerns into the hands of God. These times under-score the importance of practicing surrender and relying on God's guidance and provision, especially when circumstances feel overwhelming.

Spiritual Dryness: Stress can create a sense of spiritual dryness—a feeling of distance from God's presence. The weight of stressors might lead you to feel isolated or abandoned in your struggles.

Questioning God's Goodness: Stressful situations may prompt questions about God's goodness and love. We might wonder why God allows hard-ships, leading to internal conflicts between our beliefs and our experiences.

The 3-Step Reset

> *"Cast all your anxiety on him because he cares for you."* (1 Peter 5:7 NIV)

So what's the solution?

My goal is to give you a new perspective on stress management so that it's not just a luxury or merely about finding moments of tranquility, but about optimizing your body's functions to support effective weight release.

Managing your stress levels is the biggest of our Core Four ways to maximize your energy, so it's imperative that you learn how to incorporate it into your daily lifestyle.

In my online *Weight Loss, God's Way* program (weightlossgodsway.com), we equip ourselves with powerful tools to effectively address stress that show up both in our lives as well as those that often accompany the weight loss journey. Among these tools, one of the most significant is the practice of our 3-Step Reset.

I'm excited to share this with you because it is our steadfast companion throughout our *Weight Loss, God's Way* program.

Picture this: You're wrestling with emotional eating, standing at the crossroads of temptation, grappling with consuming fears, having a heated argument, dealing with work stress or spiraling down a rabbit hole of negative thoughts. In these moments, the 3-Step Reset emerges as your steadfast ally—offering clarity, strength, and a pathway forward.

It's elegantly simple, yet profoundly effective—a tool that empowers you to reclaim control, regain focus, and realign with your God-given purpose. As we journey together, you'll discover the various facets of this reset and witness its transformative impact on your life. The 3-Step Reset is composed of the pause, pray, and practice.

"He says, 'Be still, and know that I am God.'" (Psalms 46:10 NIV)

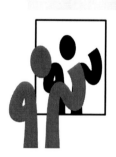

Step 1. The Pause: A Moment of Intentional Awareness

In John Eldredge's book *Get Your Life Back*, the importance of the 'pause' is a central theme. Eldredge emphasizes that in our fast-paced digital age, taking regular pauses is crucial for our mental, emotional, and spiritual well-being.

The Pause allows us to break free from the constant noise and distractions of modern life, providing a space for reflection, connection with God, and self-care. It enables us to regain a sense of perspective, find peace amidst chaos, and nurture our inner lives.

The Pause doesn't merely mean to 'stop'; it's a moment of intentional awareness. It's that crucial moment when you slow down, step out of the chaotic whirlwind of life, and pay attention to what's happening within you. This pause is multi-dimensional, encompassing various aspects of your being:

Physical Awareness. The Pause prompts you to tune in to your physical body. It's about noticing the subtle cues it sends—perhaps a racing heart, a pang of hunger, or a surge of energy. By doing so, you foster a deeper connection with your body's needs and responses.

Mental Clarity. In the realm of thoughts, the Pause is your sanctuary. It's the space where you take a step back and observe your own thinking patterns. Are you entertaining thoughts of quitting? Are you besieged by doubts? This mental pause helps you gain clarity and insight into the thoughts that might be leading you astray.

Emotional Exploration. Emotions can often steer us off course. The Pause encourages you to dig into your emotional landscape. It might reveal feelings of fear, restlessness, or the desire to escape. By acknowledging these emotions, you begin to understand their role in your weight releasing journey.

Spiritual Alignment. At its core, the Pause is about spiritual alignment. It's the moment when you tune in to the voice of God, the divine promptings that guide you. This spiritual pause enables you to seek God's wisdom, align your spirit with His, and find the strength to continue on your path.

The Calming and Realignment Effect

Now, let's explore why this pause is so vital.

Pausing calms your nervous system. In times of stress, your nervous system can become overstimulated and frazzled. The Pause serves as a reset button for your nervous system. It's a calming breath, a moment of stillness that soothes the stress and restores balance.

It realigns body, soul, and spirit. Your being consists of body, soul, and spirit, intricately interconnected. The Pause is the thread that weaves them together in harmony. It realigns your body with your soul and spirit, creating a synergy that empowers you to move forward with purpose.

The wisdom of Psalms 46:10 echoes through the Pause. In stillness you find clarity, divine guidance, and the wisdom that flows from the Holy Spirit. It's in this tranquil moment where you can decipher the noise of the world from the whispers of God.

It unmasks limiting thoughts and beliefs. Without the Pause, limiting thoughts often lurk in the shadows of your subconscious mind. They silently influence your actions and choices. However, when you pause and pay attention, these thoughts are brought into the light of your conscious mind. This awareness is the first step in dismantling their power over you.

The Art of Pausing: A Simple Guide

Isn't it crazy that in our busy lives pausing can feel like a luxury we can't afford? Yet it's precisely when life gets hectic that we need to take a step back and regain our sense of balance.

How to Pause: The Box Breathing Technique

One of the most effective ways to pause and center yourself is through the practice of box breathing. It's a simple yet powerful technique that can be done anywhere, anytime, and it only takes a few minutes. Here's how to do it:

Find A Quiet Space: If possible, choose a quiet spot where you won't be disturbed. However, you can practice this technique even in the midst of a busy day.

Get Comfortable: Sit in a comfortable position with your back straight. You can also stand if that's more comfortable for you.

The 5-5-5-5 Pattern:

Inhale: Close your eyes and take a slow, deep breath in through your nose for a count of 5. Feel the air filling your lungs and expanding your chest.

Hold: Hold your breath for another count of 5. This is a moment of stillness where you can center your thoughts and focus inward.

Exhale: Slowly exhale through your mouth for a count of 5, releasing any tension or stress.

Pause: After exhaling, pause for a final count of 5. During this moment, simply be present and acknowledge the presence of God.

As you practice box breathing, use this time to connect with God. Smile and recognize His presence in your life. You can express your gratitude for His love, guidance, and the opportunity to pause and reflect.

Remember that pausing is a skill that can be cultivated over time. Initially, you might find it challenging to capture your racing thoughts or fully immerse yourself in the pause. That's okay, it's all part of the process. Be patient with yourself, and with practice you'll become more adept at pausing and finding stillness amidst life's chaos.

In the chapters ahead, we'll explore more ways to integrate the art of pausing into your daily routine. It's a valuable tool that will help you navigate your emotions, overcome temptations, and stay aligned with your spiritual journey. As you practice the Pause, you'll discover the impact it has on your overall well-being and your connection with God.

Step 2. Pray: Communing with God

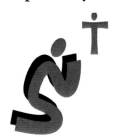

Now that you understand the power of the Pause, let's move on to the second step in our 3-Step Reset: Prayer.

Why Prayer?

If you're familiar with the story of David and Goliath, you'll remember that it was David's faith in the Lord Almighty that allowed him to bring down such a mighty giant. We, too, are confronted daily with our own giants—whether it's the temptation to overeat, emotional triggers, or self-doubt. Our human strength alone is no match for these formidable opponents. It's time to recognize that we have been equipped with powerful spiritual weapons by God Himself.

> *1 Samuel 17:45 (NIV) says, "David said to the Philistine,*
> *'You come against me with sword and spear and javelin, but*
> *I come against you in the name of the LORD Almighty, the*
> *God of the armies of Israel.'"*

David's trust in the Lord was his ultimate weapon, and it's a lesson we can apply to our own battles. When it comes to overcoming strongholds like overeating, emotional struggles, or the allure of innutritious foods, our own efforts may feel like bringing a knife to a gunfight—ineffective and powerless. However, God has provided us with divine artillery, including prayer, His Word, and the Holy Spirit. These are the tools we need to dismantle every obstacle that stands in the way of our relationship with Him.

The Many Forms of Prayer

Your prayer during this step can take various forms, depending on the situation you're facing:

1. Traditional Prayer. This is the classic conversation with God, where you lay your concerns, fears, or desires before Him. It can be as simple as, "Lord, give me strength to resist this temptation", or "Guide me through this challenging moment".

2. Declaration. Sometimes you need to assert your faith and authority. You can declare, "I am more than a conqueror through Christ who strengthens me", or "I am free from the power of emotional eating".

3. Confession. Acknowledge your need for God's intervention and confess your reliance on His strength. Say, "I can't do this alone, Lord. I need Your help to overcome this struggle".

The type of prayer you choose depends on the situation and your personal connection with God. There's no one-size-fits-all approach. It's about cultivating a prayer life that aligns with your unique journey.

Once you've paused, incorporate one of the forms of prayer into the situation you're facing. Remember that prayer isn't just a last resort—it's your first line of defense in your weight releasing journey. By inviting God into every aspect of your life, including your health and well-being, you tap into a wellspring of divine strength that empowers you to overcome any obstacle.

> *"The weapons we fight with are not the weapons of the world. On the contrary, they have divine power to demolish strongholds." (2 Corinthians 10:4 NIV)*

Step 3: Practice – The Power of Active Practice

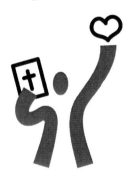

Now that we've explored the first two steps of our 3-Step Reset—pausing and praying—it's time to discover the third and equally essential step: Practice. As we venture into this phase, remember the significance of each preceding step. You've already cultivated awareness by pausing and inviting God's strength through prayer.

Step 3 introduces the concept of 'Active Practice'—a dynamic tool that helps you to retrain your mind and transform unhealthy thought patterns.

In both Biblical and modern contexts, specific actions, gestures, movements, or postures hold practical purposes and symbolic meanings. Consider David's raised hands in prayer (Psalms 63:4), Moses and Joshua removing their shoes on holy ground (Exodus 3:5), or Jeremiah placing stones in a brick kiln (Jeremiah 43:8–13).

Even in your life today, you may engage in gestures like clapping to express gratitude or snapping an elastic band on your wrist to shift negative behavior. These actions have the potential to enhance memory, facilitate learning, solve problems, and improve communication.

The Power of Active Practice

'Active Practice' is a potent tool to retrain your brain and create healthy thoughts.

The concept of 'Active Practice' is not only rooted in spiritual and psychological principles, but is also supported by scientific insights into how the human mind works.

Here are a few of them:

One of the key scientific foundations of 'Active Practice' is neuroplasticity—the brain's remarkable ability to adapt, change, and rewire itself in response to learning and experience. When you engage in active practices repeatedly, you're essentially carving new neural pathways in your brain. This process allows you to replace old, unhealthy thought patterns with new, positive ones. The more you practice the stronger these neural connections become, making it easier to default to healthier thinking over time.

It also serves as a form of positive reinforcement. When you engage in these actions in response to unhealthy thoughts, you're providing your brain with a rewarding experience. This positive feedback loop reinforces the idea that replacing unhealthy thoughts with positive actions leads to a sense of accomplishment and satisfaction, encouraging you to continue these practices.

Active practices like taking slow, deep breaths or engaging in physical movement have been scientifically proven to regulate emotions. Deep breathing, for example, activates the parasympathetic nervous system, which counteracts the 'fight or flight' response and induces a state of calmness. By incorporating such practices, you can effectively manage emotional reactions triggered by negative thoughts.

Certain active practices can enhance memory and facilitate learning. When you pair an active practice with prayer, a specific declaration or positive affirmation, you create an association that reinforces memory recall. This can be particularly helpful in situations where you need to remember and apply these affirmations in real-time, such as when confronted with an unhealthy thought. For example, placing your hand over your heart whenever you're tempted by unhealthy food choices, your affirmation is, "I honor my body as God's temple by nourishing it with wholesome foods." Over time this repetition will reinforce your ability to choose healthier options consistently, contributing to your overall success in managing your weight.

Lastly, many active practices such as clapping or stomping your feet strengthen the mind-body connection. This connection plays a vital role in emotional regulation and overall well-being. As you practice 'Active Practice' you become more attuned to the sensations in your body, allowing you to recognize and address negative thought patterns as they arise.

I hope that by understanding the science behind these practices you can approach them with confidence, knowing that they are grounded in both spiritual as well as evidence-based strategies for your breakthrough.

Now it's time to select your Active Practice. You can opt for a single active practice to repeat daily as you progress through this book, or you can choose different ones based on the specific toxic thoughts you encounter.

In the coming chapters you'll have opportunities to practice it, but for now here are some examples.

1. Take a Step Forward: Symbolizing your departure from the past, a step forward signifies your movement towards a healthier mindset and future.

2. Hands Over Your Heart: This gesture reflects the deep love God has for you. Placing your hands over your heart serves as a reminder of His unconditional love.

3. Stomp Your Feet: Visualize yourself stomping on the toxic thought, forcefully removing it from your life, and replacing it with a positive perspective.

4. Exalt the Name of the Lord: Lift your voice and exalt God's Name, acknowledging His sovereignty and drawing strength from His presence.

5. Smile and Visualize: With a smile on your face, picture God's pleasure in you and visualize His joy surrounding your life.

6. Hands Lifted in Surrender: This posture signifies surrender to God's guidance, trusting in His plan for your transformation.

7. Clap in Victory: Celebrate your victory over negative thoughts with a hearty clap. This action reinforces your commitment to a positive mindset.

8. Sing a Verse of a Related Song: Singing a verse from a meaningful song can help reinforce positive thoughts and redirect your focus.

9. Draw or Sketch Something: Engaging your creative side by drawing or sketching can be a therapeutic way to channel your thoughts.

10. Visualize Jesus Beside You: Envision Jesus sitting beside you, offering His unwavering support and guidance on your journey.

These are just a few examples of active practices that you can incorporate into your daily routine. Choose the ones that resonate with you the most, and as you practice them consistently, you'll find them becoming powerful tools in your weight releasing toolkit.

> *"I will praise you as long as I live, and in your name I will lift up my hands." (Psalms 63:4 NIV)*

Now let's go back to our conversation about stress management. So how would you use the 3-Step Reset to help you?

Here are three examples of how to use the 3-Step Reset to help calm stress levels so you can maximize your energy and effectively steward your temple.

Emotional Eating:

Pause. Recognize the stressful situation or emotional trigger that's causing you to consider unhealthy eating choices. Pause and take a deep breath to acknowledge the stress and the temptation.

Pray. Offer a brief prayer to seek God's strength and guidance in this moment. You might say, "Lord, I'm feeling stressed, and I need Your help to make a healthy choice right now."

Practice. Implement an 'Active Practice' of placing your hand over your heart and repeat an affirmation like, "I choose to honor my body with nourishing food."

Workplace Stress:

Pause. When you encounter a stressful situation at work, such as a demanding project or a difficult coworker, pause for a moment. Acknowledge the stress without judgment.

Pray. Offer a quick prayer for wisdom and patience. You might say, "Lord, grant me the wisdom to handle this situation calmly and the patience to work through it effectively."

Practice. Choose an 'Active Practice' like taking a step back from your desk or workspace, closing your eyes briefly, and taking a few deep breaths. As you do this, visualize yourself overcoming the stressor and finding a solution. This practice can help you return to your tasks with a calmer mindset.

Family Conflict:

Pause. In the midst of a heated argument or family tension, pause and take a moment to recognize your emotions. This might only be 5-10 seconds depending on the situation.

Pray. Pray for peace and understanding in the family. Ask for guidance in handling the situation with love and patience. You might say, "Lord, help us find common ground and resolve our differences with love."

Practice. Your chosen 'Active Practice' could involve clasping your hands together symbolizing unity while repeating a declaration (in your head) like, "I surrender this conversation to You, Lord, and I choose love and understanding."

In all these scenarios, the 3-Step Reset helps you manage stress by introducing a deliberate pause, inviting God's presence and guidance through prayer instead of holding on to the tension and anxiety, and using an 'Active Practice' to redirect your thoughts and actions. This approach empowers you to respond to stressors with more composure and make healthier choices, whether in your eating habits or in handling challenging situations.

In this chapter, you discovered a counter approach to stress and weight releasing. Instead of resisting and struggling in your own strength, you learned to shift your mindset towards letting go and releasing. This change in perspective not only makes the journey more enjoyable, but also sustainable. When faced with stress in our health journey, I encourage you to question if there's something you're trying to resist and release it to God using the 3-Step Reset. This newfound perspective allows you to approach your health and weight goals with enthusiasm, relying on God's strength and guidance for a successful and fulfilling journey.

Principle 3 Summary

Reflect on these key points:

- "What you resist persists and what you release flows with ease." The very act of trying to lose weight leads to stress, anxiety, and consequently weight gain.

- Stress management isn't just a luxury, but a crucial component of our journey towards releasing excess weight and embracing a healthier lifestyle.

- Practice the 3-Step Reset to help you manage stress.

Principle #4: Change Your Relationship with Food

Ditch the Diets

If you're anything like me, food has played a significant role in your life. And if like me you've been on a dieting journey for an extended period, it may have consumed unhealthy amounts of your time and energy. I still recall my initial attempt at dieting when I was around 12 years old which, rather regrettably, consisted of a steady intake of laxatives. It wasn't a 'real' diet, but it shows the extremes that I and countless others like me have gone to in pursuit of a healthier weight.

Despite how much attention we give to food, we are none the wiser about how to stop ourselves from the lure of overconsumption of unhealthy foods, or how we're to eat to maintain a healthy weight once we have achieved it.

It's enough for us to want to surrender with the white flag and say, "Pass the Häagen-Dazs!"

We're so busy trying to figure out calories, points, and the latest low-carb foods that it allows the enemy to have a field day with us. He's won again by keeping us distracted and focusing on minutiae that were never meant to take up so much of our time.

We've made food a mystery to be solved—a puzzle to be pieced together and a vault to be entered into with a magical combination—but it's so much more than any of these approaches. Often, food is viewed as either the adversary, hindering our ability to relish life, or conversely as our ally. A companion during moments of joy and a source of comfort in times of sorrow. It has been our reward for achievements and our solace in times of stress.

I am committed to helping you break down your old beliefs about food so that you can erect a new Biblical and holistic approach to your health.

Traditionally, weight loss has centered around cutting your calories or eliminating certain food groups like carbohydrates or fats. Unfortunately, like we learned in the last chapter on stress management, this approach can often have the opposite effect.

Restriction and Deprivation. Labeling certain foods as "off-limits" or "bad" leads to restrictive eating patterns and deprivation, which are common features of diets. We may go on a strict diet, cutting out entire food groups or severely limiting our calorie intake. This restriction can lead to short-term weight loss but is difficult to maintain in the long run, leading to a cycle of dieting and overeating.

Emotional Eating. Many people with an unhealthy relationship with food use it as a coping mechanism for stress, emotions, or boredom. This emotional eating can lead to overconsumption of comfort foods, followed by guilt and the desire to go on a diet to "undo" the damage. This perpetuates the diet mindset as we constantly swing between emotional eating and strict dieting. We'll talk more about this in the chapter on developing emotional resilience.

All-or-Nothing Thinking. Restricting caloric intake often encourages all-or-nothing thinking, where we are either "on" the diet or "off" the diet. This binary mindset can be damaging because it doesn't allow for flexibility or moderation. It makes you a slave to food. When we inevitably deviate from the diet, we may feel like we've failed and return to old eating habits, reinforcing the dieting cycle.

Negative Self-Image. Restricting caloric intake often promises rapid weight loss and a transformed body. However, these promises can create unrealistic body image expectations. When we don't achieve these idealized results quickly, we may become discouraged and feel negatively about our bodies. This negative self-image can perpetuate the diet mindset as we continue to seek the next quick fix.

Short-Term Focus. Restricting calories tends to focus on short-term goals, such as shedding a certain number of pounds in a few weeks. This short-term focus can lead to a "quick fix" mentality, where we prioritize immediate weight loss over long-term health and sustainable habits. When the diet ends, we may return to our old habits and regain the lost weight.

External Validation. Having a dieting mindset often relies on external validation, such as the number on the scale or the opinions of others, to measure success. This external focus can disconnect us from our internal cues of hunger and fullness, making it difficult to develop a healthy and intuitive relationship with food. It can also deafen us to hearing God's voice as He leads and guides us.

Lower Your Body's Set Point. When you consistently consume fewer calories than your body requires for its basic functions and activity level, your metabolism can slow down to conserve energy. This adaptation is a survival mechanism designed to prevent excessive weight loss. As your metabolism slows, your body becomes more efficient at using the calories you do consume, making weight loss more difficult.

Hormonal Changes. Calorie restriction can lead to changes in hormonal levels, particularly hormones like leptin and ghrelin, which regulate hunger and fullness. When you eat fewer calories, your body may produce less leptin (the hormone that signals fullness) and more ghrelin (the hormone that stimulates hunger). This hormonal imbalance can increase appetite and make it harder to maintain a reduced calorie intake.

Muscle Loss. Severe calorie restriction can lead to the loss of lean muscle mass. Muscle tissue burns more calories at rest than fat tissue, so when you lose muscle your resting metabolic rate decreases. This can further lower your calorie expenditure and contribute to weight regain.

Plateau Effect. Over time, your body may adapt to a lower calorie intake by becoming more efficient at using the available energy. This adaptation can create a plateau in weight loss, making it challenging to continue losing weight despite continued calorie restriction.

I hope I've provided you with ample reasons to bid farewell to diets and wholeheartedly embrace a new, sustainable approach to your health and well-being. It's time to move away from the cycle of restrictive eating and welcome a journey that nourishes your body, mind, and soul. By doing so, you can discover a path that not only leads to a healthier weight but also fosters lasting vitality, freedom, and joy in your life.

Food as Favor, Fulfillment, and Fuel

I hope it's now clearer why trying to lose weight by cutting calories may have posed such a challenge for you in the past. It's like fighting a battle against your own body when you engage in calorie restriction. My intention is for this realization to serve as a wake-up call, prompting you to bid farewell to the dieting cycle once and for all.

Now that you understand why conventional diets often fall short, let's shift our focus to a fresh perspective—one that empowers you to approach your health and weight goals in a more sustainable and holistic manner.

The goal is to move away from **DIE**TS TO **HEAL**TH. Did you catch that? We want to learn to eat to heal, fuel, and nourish our bodies instead of eating foods that lead to our slow death. This comes back to eating foods to maximize your energy.

Here are the three shifts in perspective you will need to make if you want to develop a healthier relationship with food.

1. Food as Favor (A Gift of God)

In my Weight Loss God's Way program, we firmly believe that food is a divine gift from God. When you view food as a favor, you are acknowledging it as an expression of His love, grace, and provision.

Consider Psalms 136:25 NIV:

> *"He gives food to every creature. His love endures forever."*

This verse reminds you that God's love is intertwined with the act of providing sustenance to all living beings. Food is not merely a means of survival; it is an extension of God's enduring love. Just as He cared for the Israelites during their sojourn in the wilderness, providing them with manna from heaven, His love continues to manifest in the nourishment you receive each day.

This perspective encourages you to approach your meals with deep gratitude and reverence. You learn to savor the flavors, colors, and textures of the foods you consume, recognizing that they are more than just nutrients—they are a manifestation of God's boundless love and care for you. When you see food as a favor, it transforms your relationship with it into a sacred act of nourishment and gratitude.

Imagine sitting down to a meal, and before you take a single bite you pause to reflect on the grace and love infused into every morsel. Your plate becomes a sacred offering, and your gratitude flows from a heart attuned to God's abundant provision. In this moment you savor not only the flavors, colors, and textures of your food but also the deeper connection to the Creator who sustains you.

As you cultivate this perspective of food as a divine favor, your relationship with nourishment deepens. Each meal becomes an act of communion with God, a tangible reminder of His ever-present love. Gratitude infuses your daily life, transforming the ordinary into the extraordinary. You begin to view food not as a mere necessity but as a sacred gift, and this shift in perspective becomes a catalyst for change on your journey to health and wellness.

In the simplest act of breaking bread you recognize the simple truth that God's love endures forever, and it is woven into the very fabric of your existence, sustaining your body and soul. With every bite you taste the sweetness of His grace, and with every meal you celebrate the divine favor that is abundantly bestowed upon you.

2. Food as Fulfillment (A Source of Enjoyment)

God, in His infinite wisdom and love, has granted you the extraordinary gift of taste buds and the ability to derive pleasure from the act of eating. Consider reshaping your connection with food, perceiving it as a sacred opportunity to discover fulfillment and joy in the nourishment you partake in.

Psalms 34:8 NIV says: *"Taste and see that the Lord is good; blessed is the one who takes refuge in Him."* These words resonate deeply with the idea that tasting and enjoying the flavors of the world is not only permissible but also a blessing. God has created a vast and diverse array of foods, each with its unique tastes and textures, waiting to be explored and appreciated.

Embracing food as a source of fulfillment allows you to savor every bite without the constant burden of guilt. It liberates you from the shackles of restrictive diets and invites you to celebrate the richness of God's creation. When you view food through the lens of enjoyment, your mealtime transforms into a joyful and satisfying experience, a true celebration of God's abundance.

Imagine relishing the vibrant colors of fresh fruits and vegetables, delighting in the rich flavors of wholesome grains and lean proteins, and savoring the comfort of a warm, homemade meal shared with loved ones. How can you add more of these foods to your healthy eating plan?

Be Additive

Instead of viewing your dietary choices through a lens of restriction and deprivation, why not adopt the principle of being additive. This new perspective will encourage you to see food as a source of fulfillment and nourishment rather than something to be avoided or limited. The concept is simple yet powerful: rather than focusing on what you should cut out of your diet, ask yourself, "How can I add more of these nourishing foods into my daily routine?" This shift in mindset aligns with the way your brain naturally functions.

Our brains are wired to favor addition over subtraction. Remember what you learned in the last chapter, "What you focus on expands". When we think about adding healthier choices to our meals, it creates a sense of abundance and satisfaction. On the contrary, a focus on deprivation and restriction can trigger feelings of scarcity and lead to cravings and overindulgence. By adopting the "be additive" approach, you make healthy eating more appealing and sustainable.

I hope this perspective will also empower you to explore new and nutritious foods, experiment with recipes, and gradually replace less nutritious options with better ones. It also encourages mindfulness about what you're putting into your body as you become more attuned to the foods that make you feel vibrant and energized. As you add more nourishing foods into your daily routine, you naturally crowd out the less nutritious choices, making room for a healthier, more fulfilling way of eating. Remember that God's intention is for you to experience the fullness of life, and that includes the joy of eating. Taste and see that the Lord's creation is good, and in doing so you bless yourself with the gift of fulfillment through food.

3. Food as Fuel (Nourishment and Energy Maximization)

While food provides enjoyment, it also serves as your primary source of nourishment and energy. Every bite you take is an opportunity to nourish your body, providing it with the nutrients you need to function optimally. By focusing on the nourishing aspect of food, you can make mindful choices that support your overall well-being.

This perspective encourages you to choose nutritious foods that fuel your body, enhance your vitality, and enable you to lead an active and fulfilling life. In essence, food becomes a means to maximize your energy, allowing you to better serve your God-given purposes.

1 Corinthians 10:31: *"So, whether you eat or drink, or whatever you do, do all to the glory of God,"* reminds us that our relationship with food should be a reflection of our devotion to God. When we approach eating with gratitude and reverence, seeing food as a divine gift from God (Food as Favor), we honor Him in our choices. We also honor God when we embrace the enjoyment of food (Food as Fulfillment) as a part of His abundant creation.

And when you view food as a means to nourish and maximize your energy (Food as Fuel), you acknowledge that your body is a temple of the Holy Spirit (1 Corinthians 6:19-20). Therefore, taking care of your bodies and making mindful, healthy choices becomes a form of worship! You are honoring God's design by treating your body with respect and providing it with what it needs to effectively carry out your God-given purposes with freedom, peace, and joy.

Foods that Maximize Your Energy

So you're ready to embrace this new paradigm, but you might still be wondering, *"So, what am I supposed to eat then?"* I've got you covered, but not in the way you might think. While most people seek a strict meal plan to follow, my nearly 40 years in the health industry have taught me that the perfect meal plan rarely works.

What truly proves effective is gaining an understanding of healthy eating principles that optimize your energy levels. This is where our 12 healthy eating pillars serve as practical guidelines for adopting a healthy eating approach. While we can't delve into exhaustive detail within this book as we do in our program, here's a concise overview of our pillars. Notice that we've put them through our energy evaluator so that you can approach healthy eating from a place of curiosity instead of guilt or shame.

1. Energy Evaluator: Is my food choice maximizing whole foods and minimizing processed sugars, fast foods, junk food, and unhealthy fats to maximize my energy?

   When choosing foods, prioritize products with shorter ingredient lists and fewer unpronounceable additives, focusing on whole, real foods. When you can prioritize high amounts of fiber and protein into your meals you will rarely go wrong.

2. Energy Evaluator: Does this meal incorporate a variety of foods to optimize the nutrients to maximize my energy?

   Ensure that your meals include proteins, carbohydrates, and healthy fats for a balanced intake of nutrients.

3. Energy Evaluator: Is my caloric intake aligned with my daily activity level and health goals to maximize my energy?

   Recognize that your caloric needs may vary based on your activity level, age, and health goals. Consult with a healthcare professional to determine your specific caloric requirements.

4. Energy Evaluator: Am I eating only when I'm truly hungry to maximize my energy?

   Avoid emotional eating and mindless snacking by recognizing true physical hunger and eating accordingly.

5. Energy Evaluator: Am I adapting my diet to meet my changing nutritional requirements as I age to maximize my energy?

   Pay attention to your body's cues and consider age-specific dietary adjustments with the guidance of healthcare professionals.

6. Energy Evaluator: Am I practicing mindful eating to maximize my energy?

    Eating mindfully involves savoring each bite, paying attention to flavors and textures, and eating slowly without distractions. This practice can improve digestion, control portion sizes, and promote weight management.

7. Energy Evaluator: Am I giving thanks for everything I eat to maximize my energy?

    Cultivate gratitude for the nourishment your food provides, recognizing that food is a gift from God. Offer thanks before each meal to enhance your connection to your food.

8. Energy Evaluator: Am I making balanced choices that leave me feeling satisfied and nourished to maximize my energy?

    Understand that healthy eating is not about deprivation or starvation but making intentional choices for health.

9. Energy Evaluator: Am I practicing fasting to maximize my energy?

    Explore the various types of fasting, both spiritual and nutritional, to understand how they can benefit your journey.

10. Energy Evaluator: Am I drinking enough water to maximize my energy?

    Remember that staying hydrated is crucial for overall health and weight management.

11. Energy Evaluator: Is my approach to food filled with joy and appreciation to maximize my energy?

    Follow the 80/20 rule for balance and enjoyment, understanding that food is a gift meant to be savored and celebrated. Avoid demonizing or vilifying food and find joy in the nourishment it provides.

12. Energy Evaluator: Does this food choice maximize my energy?

    Consider whether the food is a simple whole food, like fresh fruits, vegetables, whole grains, lean proteins, and nuts. Avoid artificially low-fat or low-carb options and foods that are heavily processed.

We've explored the "Energy Evaluator" to guide your choices and nourish your body and spirit. These questions will empower you to make food decisions that prioritize your energy over weight loss and being additive over depriving yourself, which will set you up for success. By considering factors such as the quality of your food, mindful eating, and adapting your eating plan to your evolving nutritional needs, you'll not only boost your energy but also naturally support your body in finding its healthy weight.

Principle 4 Summary

Reflect on these key points:

- Traditional dieting can actually have the opposite effect. You can end up gaining weight.

- Reframe food as favor, fulfillment, and fuel.

- Follow the 12 Healthy Eating Energy Evaluator questions to help inform your choices about what you should eat.

- When deciding what to eat, always prioritize energy management and being additive.

Principle #5: Move Your Body

Motion is Lotion

In the last chapter, you reframed your perspective on food. You recognized that you may have viewed food as either the adversary, hindering your ability to relish life, or conversely, as your ally—a companion during moments of joy and a source of comfort in times of sorrow. You gained a new perspective so that you can begin to see food as favor, fulfillment, and fuel. Lastly, you prioritized maximizing your energy and being additive in your food choices.

Today, you'll learn the third part of the Core Four: Physical Activity. Similar to healthy eating, this will require a possible shift in the way you've been perceiving exercise.

So how do you perceive exercise? Is it a necessary evil? Punishment for over-indulging? Something you should do? Is it a tiresome chore, a time-consuming obligation, or even a source of physical discomfort? Conversely, exercise might be your "get-out-of-jail-free" card that you use to excuse yourself from eating vast amounts of food. For me, I fell in this last category. Wherever you find yourself, these negative perspectives will hinder your motivation to engage in regular physical activity.

It's not totally your fault, though. Our natural disposition is to conserve energy, which means we're not naturally motivated to exercise. Our ancestors were wired to conserve energy for survival, so the modern concept of regular exercise can often clash with this inherent tendency. But that was never God's original intent for us. He designed our muscles, cardiovascular system, circulatory system, and nervous system to all be fueled by regular physical activity.

Have you ever heard the expression motion is lotion? It means that staying active, like applying lotion to the skin, helps keep the body functioning smoothly and reduces stiffness and discomfort.

Our bodies function optimally when we move regularly and exercise becomes an essential part of our overall well-being. It's a way to honor the magnificent creation God designed, ensuring that we maintain our health and vitality for the journey He has set before us. While it may feel like a battle against our natural instincts, embracing regular exercise aligns us with God's intended design for our bodies and enhances our physical, mental, and spiritual well-being.

I am committed to helping you break down your old beliefs about health so that you can erect a new Biblical and holistic approach to your health. In order to do that, you should understand how your current mindset about physical activity is currently sabotaging you.

Physical activity plays a crucial role in helping you release weight through various mechanisms:

Faster Weight Release: Exercise contributes to creating a calorie deficit by burning additional calories, which accelerates weight loss. Without exercise, you may need to rely solely on caloric restriction through diet, leading to a slower rate of weight loss.

Muscle Maintenance: When releasing weight, especially through diet alone, there's a risk of losing lean muscle mass along with fat. Exercise, particularly resistance training, helps preserve and build muscle, ensuring that the majority of your weight loss comes from fat rather than muscle.

Increased Metabolism: A lack of exercise can result in a decreased metabolic rate over time. This makes it easier to regain weight once you've achieved your weight release goals, as your body becomes more efficient at conserving energy.

Increased Energy and Vitality: Sedentary lifestyles can lead to feelings of constant fatigue and lethargy. Without the energy-boosting effects of exercise, you may struggle to stay alert and focused throughout the day.

Mood and Emotional Well-Being: Physical activity is known to release endorphins, which are natural mood boosters. Without regular exercise, you may be more susceptible to mood swings, anxiety, and depression.

Enhanced Sleep Quality: Regular physical activity has been shown to improve sleep quality and help with falling asleep faster. Without exercise, you may experience difficulties falling asleep, staying asleep, or achieving restorative sleep.

Even small amounts of physical activity can make a significant difference in your energy levels and overall health. Later we'll talk about simple ways that you can begin to incorporate more physical activity into your daily lifestyle.

Exercise as Worship

We've discussed how your current perception of physical activity can be contributing to your weight challenges. You might be currently viewing it as a necessary evil; punishment for overindulging; something you should do; or maybe you see it as a tiresome chore, a time-consuming obligation, or even a source of physical discomfort.

Our goal is to give you a new perspective of physical activity so you can associate it with a life of peace, ease, joy, and freedom.

Physical activity is one of the Core Four ways to maximize your energy, so it's imperative that you learn how to incorporate it into your daily lifestyle.

Here are small shifts that will have a major impact on the way you perceive physical activity.

1. See exercise as a form of worship to God.

For many of us, exercise often evokes thoughts of discomfort, tedium, and a drain on our time. Have you ever thought about how God views your efforts to care for your body through physical activity? It's not about the sweat or the time spent; it's about recognizing that every step, every lift, and every stretch can be an act of worship.

Imagine exercise as a form of worship to God. This means that every time you engage in physical activity, you are honoring the body He has entrusted to you. Your body is a sacred vessel, a temple of the Holy Spirit, as the Bible teaches. So, when you work on keeping it healthy, you are also working on your spiritual well-being.

This shift in thinking makes exercise more than just a means to an end; it becomes a meaningful part of not only your health journey but your entire life. It shifts the narrative from a burden to a blessing, from discomfort to dedication. It encourages you to appreciate every moment you spend caring for your body, whether it's a brisk walk, a stretching session, or lifting weights.

2. Create a praise playlist.

Make a connection between exercise and praise by crafting a playlist that fuels your inspiration and motivation. Utilize tracks like Mandisa's 'Overcomer' and 'Good Morning' to infuse you with energy and to reiterate that moving your body is a privilege to be cherished. Moreover, scientific evidence supports the notion that music enhances exercise performance. With each beat, your workout becomes a form of celebration and worship.

3. See it as a time to memorize Scripture.

I went through a phase where I recited scriptures during my weightlifting sessions. With every repetition, I would proclaim verses like "I can do all things through Christ who strengthens me" for the first rep, "My body is the temple of the Holy Spirit who is in me" for the second, "Greater is He who is in me than the one who is in the world" for the third, and "When I am weak, then I am strong" for the fourth, and so on. This practice transformed my workouts into moments of spiritual affirmation. Post-workout, my body, mind, and spirit felt invigorated and renewed.

4. Always be ready.

Consider slipping into your workout attire right after waking up. Prepare your gym bag the night before to streamline your routine. Seek chances to be active throughout your day, no matter the time or place. As you start viewing exercise as an act of worship, your eagerness to engage in it will naturally grow, prompting you to make it a frequent practice.

5. Shift exercise from must-do to get-to-do.

Change the way you think about exercise—see it as something cool you get to do, not just another thing on your list. Instead of feeling like you have to do it, realize you're lucky to have the chance to move your body and take care of yourself. This shift in mindset makes exercise feel like a treat, not a chore. It's a chance to feel good and work towards your health goals, all while enjoying the process.

Let's home in on the first point, seeing exercise as worship.

> *"For in him we live, and move, and have our being."* (*Acts 17:28 NIV*)

Acts 17:28 is a reminder that your physical movements, including exercise, are part of a bigger picture of your life in God's presence. Reframing exercise as worship integrates your physical health into your spiritual journey, deepening your connection with God as you care for the temple He has provided.

When you reframe exercise as an act of worship, you recognize that every moment of your life and every time you move, you are reflecting God's glory. Without guilt or shame, see it as your reasonable service to him as Romans 12:1 teaches us.

This understanding also fosters gratitude and appreciation for the gift of a healthy body and the ability to move. When you exercise with the intention of worship, you approach it with thankfulness for the body God has provided and the opportunity to maintain and improve it.

Types of Physical Activity

Having a new perspective is good, but now it's your turn to take action.

Exercise will look different for everyone. It might entail hitting the gym for weightlifting, causing exertion and muscle strain, or it could be a leisurely stroll with a friend. Each of these constitutes a form of exercise.

This chapter will give you a comprehensive understanding of exercise and its essential components to create a holistic workout routine.

Exercise encompasses any physical activity that elevates or sustains physical fitness and overall well-being. It encompasses cardiovascular health, muscular strength, flexibility, and endurance. The activities you choose hinges on your objectives and personal inclinations. To optimize fat loss, a balanced approach usually involves dedicating more time to cardiovascular and muscular conditioning or strength training. As you age, muscular strength must be prioritized.

Cardiovascular Fitness (or aerobic exercise)

It is the ability of your heart and lungs to supply oxygen-rich blood to all the muscles in the body. It is strengthened by performing activities such as running, walking, swimming, cycling, or anything that will elevate your heart rate.

Benefits:

1. Improves cardiovascular health
2. Lowers blood pressure
3. Helps regulate blood sugar
4. Reduces asthma symptoms
5. Reduces chronic pain
6. Aids sleep
7. Regulates weight
8. Strengthens the immune system
9. Improves brain power
10. Boosts mood
11. Reduces the risk of falls

How Much Do You Need?

Around 30 minutes of moderate cardiovascular activity is <u>recommended</u> at least 5x per week.

Muscular and Conditioning (or strength training)

It is the maximum amount of force that your muscles can exert in a single maximal effort. The three most effective ways to improve your muscular strength and endurance are by using the resistance of your own body weight (such as push-ups, squats, or lunges), free weights (dumbbells), or machines. What method you choose is determined by your goals, availability of equipment, limitations due to previous injuries, and personal preferences.

Benefits:

Strong muscles will:

1. Improve your posture

2. Reduce your risk of injury

3. Make your everyday activities easier

4. Preserve muscle mass

5. Control weight

6. Reduce risk of osteoporosis

How Much Do You Need?

It is recommended to perform strength training exercises a <u>minimum of 2x per week.</u>

Flexibility (or stretching)

Is the range of motion around each of your individual joints. Flexibility is improved by stretching, which means exerting a slight amount of tension on the joints and holding it there for about 10 seconds to three minutes.

Benefits:

Flexibility helps decrease your risk of injury and muscle soreness after a workout. It helps prevent lower back pain, improves physical performance, and improves your circulation.

How Much Do You Need?

Stretching can be performed every day as long as you're not overdoing it. If you're new to stretching, you can start with just five minutes per day or 15 minutes 3x per week.

The bottom line: Good fitness involves strength and efficiency in all three areas. Overworking one area while neglecting the others can lead to problems. To maximize fat loss, your goal is to burn more calories than you consume. So begin by increasing the amount of activity you're currently performing.

Physical Activity Tips and Suggestions

I encourage clients to be focused and intense when they are exercising; however, not all of your workouts should be at the same intensity. I usually encourage one intense day, one moderate day, and one lighter day per week when doing both aerobic exercise and muscle conditioning. When all your workouts are the same high intensity, your body can get overstressed, and you can actually start to experience negative effects.

Think of your weekly routine if you have one. Are some workouts more challenging than others? If not, how can you change it up to vary the intensity?

Balance your work/rest ratio

Rest is just as important as exercising. Your body needs to rest both during your workouts and also on the days when you are not exercising.

Rest periods during your workouts are important during weight training or muscular conditioning exercises when you want to shape and tone your muscles. Studies have found that both testosterone and the growth hormone are produced in greater levels when you rest for short to moderate periods; 60 to 90 seconds between sets seems to be the agreed-upon rest time in the fitness world.

Rest periods are also important between your workout days. One of the most common questions I get asked is, "Is it okay to work out every day?"

Here is my usual response:

For cardiovascular fitness, it's okay to exercise every day, as long as you balance your workout by alternating between intense days and light days.

For muscle toning and strengthening, I recommend 48 hours between muscle groups. That means if you train your legs on Monday, then your next leg workout would be on Wednesday or later. It's okay, if not strictly necessary, to do strength training daily, as long as you alternate which muscles are being stressed.

Why rest days?

It's actually on your rest days that your muscles get stronger. On your rest days the muscles you trained get repaired and healed. If you have not had adequate rest, your body cannot regenerate itself. Without adequate rest, you run the risk of injury, you may not get the results you're looking for, and you may even see a decrease in your performance.

Balance your upper body and lower body

Do you spend as much time on your upper body as you do on your lower body? Men tend to spend more time on their upper body, especially the bench press, while women tend to spend too much time on their lower body, especially the inner and outer thigh machines. Resist the urge to focus on one or the other.

If your current routine is only walking, think about adding some hand weights or upper body exercises to your routine.

Whether it's a brisk walk, a dance session in your living room, or a few minutes of stretching, every movement counts. As you integrate exercise into your daily life, you'll not only enhance your physical health but also draw closer to the Creator who designed you. Let's wrap up this chapter with our energy evaluator. It will help you to inform your choices about not only whether you should move more, but also what type of movement will help to maximize your energy. Here are some examples of questions to ask yourself:

1. Energy Evaluator: Does engaging in an intense cardio workout maximize my energy, or would a gentle stretch session align better with my energy management goal?

This question encourages you to assess which exercise option will leave you feeling more energized and in tune with your overall well-being.

2. Energy Evaluator: How many hours have I been sitting down today?

   Here, consider how long you've been sitting down. I've heard expressions such as, "sitting is the new smoking" alluding to the dangers of sitting all day. Getting up each hour for a couple of minutes will help you to maximize your overall energy.

3. Energy Evaluator: Does taking the stairs instead of the elevator for a quick office visit enhance my energy and overall physical activity, or is using the elevator a wiser choice, considering my current energy levels?

   This question encourages you to look for alternative ways to move so that you can maximize your energy throughout the day

4. Energy Evaluator: Will engaging in a long, vigorous hike maximize my energy, or would a short, brisk walk in the park be a better choice for my overall energy goal?

   This question helps you determine which type of physical activity aligns with your goal of maximizing energy and overall well-being.

5. Energy Evaluator: Will hitting the gym after a tiring day at work revitalize my energy, or should I schedule my workout for the morning when I'm fresh and energized?

   By asking this question, you consider the timing of your workout and its impact on your energy levels, making a choice that aligns with your well-being and energy management.

6. Energy Evaluator: What can I do today to increase my energy?

   If there is not a lot of activity in your day, how can you squeeze more in? Can you turn housework into a workout? Can you bring your groceries in one bag at a time? Can you stand up while you're talking on the phone instead of sitting? Look for ways you can squeeze it in.

Principle 5 Summary

Reflect on these key points:

- Motion is Lotion. Look for ways that you can increase your movement and therefore maximize your energy.

- Reframe exercise as a form a worship; see it as your reasonable service to God as Romans 12:1 teaches.

- Physical activity should include cardiovascular exercises, strength training, and flexibility exercises.

- As you go about the day, use the energy evaluator to inform your movement choices.

Principle #6: Sleep Well

Go To Bed

Sleep, often overlooked yet highly influential, is the fourth essential component of the Core Four when it comes to maximizing your energy and stewarding your temple. It's a piece of the puzzle that many underestimate or even neglect in their pursuit of a healthier life. What might come as a surprise to you is that, even if you're diligently following a healthy lifestyle and making all the right choices in terms of nutrition and physical activity, you might still find yourself struggling with your weight if you're not getting adequate sleep.

The connection between sleep and weight management is a complex and intricate one, rooted in the intricate workings of our bodies and minds. When you don't get enough sleep, it disrupts the delicate balance of hormones and processes that regulate your appetite, metabolism, and energy expenditure.

One of the primary hormones affected is ghrelin, often referred to as the "hunger hormone". Ghrelin levels increase when you're sleep-deprived, sending powerful signals to your brain that it's time to eat. Simultaneously, insufficient sleep reduces the levels of leptin, the hormone responsible for signaling fullness and satiety. This hormonal imbalance results in an increased appetite, particularly for high-calorie, sugary, and fatty foods—the kind of foods you're more likely to indulge in when your willpower is compromised by exhaustion.

Also, lack of sleep impacts your body's ability to efficiently process and regulate blood sugar. It leads to insulin resistance, making your cells less responsive to insulin's signal to let glucose in, ultimately raising your blood sugar levels. These elevated blood sugar levels can contribute to weight gain and increase the risk of developing type 2 diabetes over time.

The consequences of sleep deprivation don't stop there. It can also sabotage your ability to make sound decisions, particularly when it comes to food choices. The prefrontal cortex, the part of your brain responsible for impulse control and decision-making, becomes impaired with insufficient sleep, leading to a greater tendency to reach for those comfort foods and sugary snacks.

Additionally, the fatigue and irritability that often accompany sleep deprivation can make it challenging to find the motivation and energy to engage in regular physical activity. Thus, a lack of sleep can indirectly impact your weight by hindering your ability to maintain an active lifestyle.

Muscle Recovery and Growth. Adequate sleep is crucial for muscle recovery and growth, especially when incorporating exercise into your weight-release journey. Quality sleep promotes the release of growth hormones supporting muscle repair and development, ultimately boosting your metabolism.

Stress and Emotional Well-Being. Insufficient sleep can amplify stress levels and negatively impact emotional well-being. Elevated stress levels can trigger emotional eating, a significant barrier to weight release.

> *"In vain you rise early and stay up late, toiling for food to eat—for he grants sleep to those he loves."* (Psalms 127:2 ESV)

How Much Sleep Do You Need?

The amount of sleep you need varies by age and by individual. A good measure of how much you need is how you feel when you wake up in the morning. If you feel refreshed and energetic, then you had a good night's sleep. The National Sleep Foundation's guidelines recommend 7–9 hours for the average adult.

Know that God has designed your body perfectly to rise feeling refreshed, be productive during the day, and rest at night. Staying up late dishonors your body. Commit to honoring God's Word and your body by accepting God's gift of rest.

In Principle 9, "Develop a System", we will discuss specific strategies to help you sleep better.

Let's close with this thought:

If God designed our bodies to sleep one-third of our lifetime, then He must want us to give it a priority in our lives.

Nowhere in life, aside from working, do we spend so much time doing one thing. Hopefully, once you understand the importance of sleep, you will value it more and give it the time and attention it rightfully deserves.

Remember, sleep is not just an innocent bystander in the world of weight management—it's an active participant. Prioritizing sleep as an integral part of your weight release strategy isn't just a luxury, it's about optimizing your body's functions for effective and sustainable progress. Remember that the power of sleep is a gift you can embrace to enhance your overall well-being and support your weight-release goals. Use the energy evaluator to help you make informed lifestyle choices.

Does this maximize my energy?

Every year, I make my pilgrimage to New York City just before Thanksgiving. The contrast between the bustling streets of the city and the serene quiet of my home in Barrie, Ontario, always strikes me. On one particular trip, I was determined to immerse myself in the city's energy. I walked tirelessly, exploring Chinatown, Little Italy, Times Square, and Central Park, absorbing every sight and sound the city had to offer. The thrill of discovery kept me on high alert, although getting lost a few times induced a touch of anxiety. Nonetheless, I pressed on, walking for nearly seven hours.

By the time I returned home, exhaustion had seeped into my body and soul. My body craved carbohydrates, my mind needed rest, and I indulged without restraint. Slumping on the couch, I mindlessly delved into six hours of binge-watching TV. But the spiral didn't end there. Snacking continued well past my eating window, leading to a drink and a reckless disregard for healthy boundaries. The morning brought a heavy food hangover, the kind that leaves your eyes swollen and your body feeling utterly depleted.

Though guilt was no longer my companion, I prayed and repented to God for dishonoring his temple. In the quiet of my soul, a simple yet profound message emerged: "Next time, just go to bed."

It struck me—the simplicity and wisdom in God's design for our bodies. It was that straightforward. My body had pleaded for rest, for sleep. Failing to heed its call, I unwittingly resorted to my old inefficient and unproductive means to sustain my energy levels. Netflix became my numbing agent, while carbohydrates acted as a quick fix for my depleted state. What I truly needed, amidst this chaotic cycle, was the simplicity of a good night's sleep.

This realization was a revelation. It uncovered the importance of sleep in our overall self-care plan. Unfortunately, the body's cry for rest often gets drowned out amidst the noise of modern living, but in its simplicity, sleep holds another key to optimal health.

How in tune are you with your body's cues for sleep? Maybe it's signaling the need for rest or heading to bed instead of trying to self-soothe using food, alcohol, TV, online shopping, or any other go-to coping mechanism. Remember, the end goal is always about maximizing your energy levels.

Consider these five practical examples for assessing, "Does this maximize my energy?", when navigating sleep-related decisions:

1. Energy Evaluator: Does staying up late to watch TV maximize my energy, or will the enjoyment be worth the potential fatigue and reduced energy levels the next day?

    This question guides you to consider the trade-off between enjoying a late-night movie and the impact it may have on your energy and overall well-being. More often than not, if you're listening, you'll hear that still, small voice telling you to go to bed.

2. Energy Evaluator: Will drinking this caffeinated or alcoholic beverage before bedtime enhance my energy management, or should I prioritize a good night's sleep over momentary stimulation?

    By asking this question, you assess whether consuming these drinks align with your goal of energy maximization or if it may hinder your sleep quality.

3. Energy Evaluator: Is it necessary to engage in a late-night work ses-

sion, or will the potential loss of sleep and increased stress negatively impact my energy and ability to perform optimally the next day?

Here, you assess whether late-night work aligns with your energy management goal and if it's worth the potential drawbacks.

4. Energy Evaluator: Will a late-night workout help me to sleep better, or is it more beneficial to opt for a gentler, earlier exercise routine that serves my energy management better?

   By asking this question, you consider whether a late-night workout is the right choice for energy maximization or if a gentler, earlier exercise routine may be more aligned with your overall well-being.

5. Energy Evaluator: Does eating this meal or snack late at night align with my overall health goals, or should I prioritize a good night's sleep over momentary stimulation?

   By asking this question, you assess whether you should sacrifice the temporary satisfaction for the potential hindrance of a good night sleep.

Principle 6 Summary

Reflect on these key points:

- Sleep can be the missing piece of the puzzle.
- Inadequate sleep impacts your hormone levels and energy levels which negatively impacts your weight.
- You need about 7-9 hours of sleep per night.
- Use the "Energy Evaluator" questions to help you prioritize sleep. In most cases, you should probably go to bed.

Principle #7: Become a Goal-Getter, not a Goal-Setter

Create S.M.A.R.T. Goals

In the first chapter, I shared my hiking journey along the Bruce Trail, drawing parallels between this expedition and your quest for health and weight release. Much like planning a hiking trip, you've set your health goals with enthusiasm and anticipation. However, you've likely encountered a familiar scenario: you plan and plan but never actually take action.

Think of goal setting as plotting the route along the Bruce Trail. You've marked your starting point and your destination, and it's clear in your mind. These goals represent your aspirations for better health, vitality, and well-being. But here's the crucial realization: having a starting point and a trail map is only the beginning. Setting out on the actual journey itself is where the real transformation occurs, and it's also where too many well-intentioned well-wishers fall short.

In the world of personal development and self-improvement, goal setting has long been celebrated as a potent tool. Every New Year, it's common practice to list ambitions, plans, and goals, fueled by the belief that this year will be different. Yet year after year, the majority of those goals fall by the wayside. It can be a soul-crushing experience to start with enthusiasm, armed with a list of well-thought-out goals, only to repeatedly fall short.

This is where our road trip analogy comes into play again. Setting goals, like planning a route on a map, is essential. It provides direction and purpose. But what's equally, if not more vital, is the journey itself. Bridging the gap between setting goals and achieving them requires a shift from mere goal setting to goal getting.

Goal setting is like casting a vision for your future—you know where you want to go, and that's an important first step. However, turning that vision into reality, like navigating blazes along the Bruce Trail, involves a more intricate process. It demands clarity, prioritizing, focus, determination, and decisive action. This shift from setting goals to getting them is another one of the keys to unlocking the transformative potential of your health and weight-releasing journey.

In this chapter, we'll explore the art of setting goals that you can genuinely achieve. In the upcoming chapters, we'll continue to build on this foundation, providing you with the tools and strategies needed to transition from a goal-setter to a goal-getter, bringing your health and weight-release aspirations to life.

It's taken me many years to understand the difference between goal-setting and goal-getting and, thankfully, you can learn the distinction right now so that you can stop frustrating yourself with setting goals that never bring you the results you seek. The process I now use and teach in our *Weight Loss, God's Way* program is the principle of S.M.A.R.T. goal setting. It stands for Specific, Measurable, Attainable, Realistic, and Time Bound.

Specific Goals

We don't achieve our goals because we often lack clarity when setting goals. Our goals are vague or lack clear definition. We might aspire to "lose weight" or "get fit", but these objectives, while well-intentioned, are not specific enough to effectively guide you. Goal getting demands precision—knowing exactly what you want and why you want it.

In the Christian community, I've also noticed that there is much confusion about whether God wants us to set specific goals or not. Some believe that 'if it's God's will' then we will do this or that, which can prevent us from taking personal responsibility for our actions by leaving it all up to God. On the other hand, some of us do the opposite and leave God out of our planning because we never thought about it or because we don't think that He really cares about this part of our lives.

Neither of these approaches is correct. The Bible offers a very balanced approach to goal setting. Luke 14:28 teaches us that we need to be specific about our plans and intentions.

> *"Suppose one of you wants to build a tower. Won't you first sit down and estimate the cost to see if you have enough money to complete it? For if you lay the foundation and are not able to finish it, everyone who sees it will ridicule you, saying, 'This person began to build and wasn't able to finish.'"* (Luke 14:28-30 NIV)

When getting specific about your goal, ask yourself the following questions:

- Is your goal well-defined?
- Does your goal line up or contradict the Word of God?
- Is your goal based on the right motive?

Here are some examples of incorrect (non-specific) goals and correct (specific) goals:

NOT SPECIFIC.

- I want to lose some weight.

SPECIFIC.

- I will release 50 pounds by December 31.
- I will walk each day.
- I will reduce my carb intake.
- I will prioritize my sleep.

Additionally, avoid trying to change too many things at once. We usually suggest changing one or two things at a time. Most people try to overhaul their entire life at once and it becomes too overwhelming, causing us to procrastinate or abandon them altogether.

Get crystal clear. Define your goals with utmost clarity. Know exactly what you want, why you want it, and how it aligns with your values and purpose. We will talk more about your values and purpose in Principle 11.

Measurable Goals

If you can't measure it, you can't manage it.

Another primary reason we struggle to achieve our health goals is our failure to track our progress effectively. The "MEASURABLE" principle in S.M.A.R.T. goal-setting underscores the significance of having clear and quantifiable criteria for evaluating our progress and overall success. It prompts us to ask whether we can effectively track and manage our goals.

Setting measurable goals ensures that your goals are specific enough to track and manage effectively. Measurement allows you to manage your goals and make necessary adjustments along the way. Just as you wouldn't embark on building a house without estimating costs and time, you shouldn't approach a weight-releasing program without specific metrics to gauge your achievements.

Here are some examples of incorrect (non-measurable) goals and correct (measurable) goals:

NOT MEASURABLE.

- I want to get in better shape.

MEASURABLE.

- I want to have a Body Mass Index of 24, and a body fat percentage of 28%. I want my blood pressure to be 125/85 and I want to be able to run five miles without stopping.

Other factors to measure to assess how you're moving toward your goal include:

1. Exercise Goal:

   How Often: I will work out five days a week.

   How Long: I plan to maintain this exercise routine for the next three months.

2. Healthy Eating Goals:

   How Much: I aim to consume five servings of vegetables and three servings of fruits daily or I will consume 1600 calories per day.

How Often: I will follow this eating pattern every day.

When: I will eat between 10:00 am to 6:00 pm every day.

3. Hydration Goal:

    How Often: I will consume at least eight glasses (64 ounces) of water every day.

    How Long: I plan to maintain this level of hydration for a minimum of three months.

4. Sleep Goal:

    How Often: I will aim for 7-8 hours of quality sleep each night.

    How Long: I will prioritize better sleep hygiene practices for the next twelve weeks.

5. Stress Management Goal:

    How Often: I will practice stress-reduction techniques (meditation, deep breathing, or the Compassion Challenge) for 15-20 minutes daily.

    How Long: I will incorporate these practices into my daily routine for the next three months.

Attainable Goals

Another significant obstacle to achieving our health goals is the tendency to set unattainable objectives. It's time to be realistic about what is and isn't possible.

It's important to recognize that there are certain aspects of ourselves that may remain relatively unchanged, no matter how hard we try. For example, if genetics dictate that you have wide hips, emulating the body shape of your favorite celebrity may be an unattainable goal. This is where aligning your goals with the Word of God becomes crucial.

By seeking alignment with God's plan for you, you can discover what is genuinely possible for your unique circumstances. It's a transformative shift from pursuing unrealistic ideals to embracing a path that aligns with God's purpose for your life. Have you ever considered asking God to reveal to you what a healthy weight looks like for you personally? This spiritual perspective can provide clarity and guidance on your journey to better health.

Here's an example of a non-attainable goal:

- Decreasing your hips to 24 inches while increasing your chest size to 38C

Here's an example of setting an attainable goal:

- Attaining a healthy BMI of 24 and waist to hip ratio of .75

> *"For I know the plans I have for you," declares the LORD, "plans to prosper you and not to harm you, plans to give you hope and a future."* (Jeremiah 29:11 NIV)

We see that whatever God has given us, it is good. We see that if we can align our goals with God's, then He will prosper us.

When you take the time to seek God, He will show you what is attainable for you. It may not be what you want, but know that it will be good.

Setting Realistic and Relevant Goals

Another common stumbling block on the path to achieving health goals is the setting of unrealistic and irrelevant objectives. It's essential to evaluate whether your goals align with your Christian values and are based on possibilities within your current lifestyle.

Goals should not only be realistic but also in harmony with your faith. What might be a realistic and healthy objective for one person could potentially lead you into sinful behavior if it pushes you to an extreme level. It's crucial to recognize that what's considered right and acceptable in the secular world may not be appropriate or in line with your Christian beliefs.

In this context, prayer and seeking wisdom are vital when setting your goals. Asking God for guidance and discernment can help ensure that your objectives are both achievable and aligned with your faith, leading to a healthier and more spiritually fulfilling journey.

Here are examples of unrealistic goals:

- I will only eat 800 calories per day until I lose weight.
- I will never eat sweets again.
- I will go to the gym every day for two hours.

Here are examples of realistic goals:

- I will eat 1500 calories per day.
- I will walk for 30 minutes per day.
- I will eat healthy 80% of the time.

Here are examples of an irrelevant goal:

- I will have my stomach stapled so I stop overeating.
- I will continue to follow the latest diet.

Here are examples of relevant goals:

- I will weigh what God wants me to weigh by learning what His plan for my health is.
- I will create a healthy meal plan based on what my body needs and choose an exercise that makes my body feel good.

> *"So I run with purpose in every step. I am not just shadow-boxing. I discipline my body like an athlete, training it to do what it should. Otherwise, I fear that after preaching to others I myself might be disqualified." (1 Corinthians 9:26-27 NLT)*

In the above scripture Paul is talking about his salvation, but we can apply the same principle here to our health. He (we) must control his (our) body and not the other way around. He (we) must train properly with focus and discipline to be successful. He (we) must prepare his (our) body the right way so that we don't disqualify ourselves.

Setting Time-Bound Goals

Another significant reason people often fail to achieve their health goals is the absence of clear timelines. Setting time-bound goals is a critical aspect of effective goal setting. This means that your goal should have both a defined start date and an end date.

The time frame you allocate to achieve your goal should strike a balance between creating a sense of urgency and being realistic. It's important that the timeline is challenging enough to inspire action but not so tight that it becomes unattainable. When you set clear deadlines your mind adjusts accordingly, and you're more likely to stay focused and motivated to accomplish your objectives.

Without a specific timeline goals can easily linger, leading to little or no progress. The absence of time-bound goals can result in procrastination and a lack of accountability, hindering your overall success in your health and weight-releasing journey.

If you've ever said to yourself, "I can't believe that I'm still here", or "I can't believe that I'm still struggling with this same issue", then you know that days, months, years, and even decades can quickly pass, and you can still find yourself in the same place.

> *"Therefore be careful how you walk, not as unwise men, but as wise, making the most of your time, because the days are evil."*
> *(Ephesians 5:15-16 NLT)*

Putting an end date on your goal does several things:

- It creates a sense of urgency.
- It helps you to create realistic timelines to work towards.
- It will keep you motivated.
- It will give you a realistic sense of the amount of effort you need to put in to achieve your goal.
- It will help you manage and schedule your time.

"So teach us to number our days. That we may gain a heart of wisdom." (Psalms 90:12 NKJV)

Unlike goal-setting, goal-getting is about taking intentional and consistent action toward your objectives. It's a dynamic approach that acknowledges the challenges and uncertainties of life while keeping you focused and committed to your intentions.

Remember that it's not just about setting the goal. It's about becoming a goal-getter. It's about turning your vision into your reality. Welcome to the journey of goal-getting—where your breakthrough awaits.

Now it's your turn! Go to breakthroughmethodbonus.com to download the free template to help you create your goal.

Understanding the Process

"Little by little I will drive them out before you until you have increased enough to take possession of the land." (Exodus 23:30 NIV)

So far you've created your vision, you understand the need to prioritize the Core Four, and you know how to go after your goals. The next crucial step in your breakthrough is to get a clearer understanding of the process of weight releasing.

Unfortunately, shows like *The Biggest Loser* would have us believe that we need to put in hours of training a day, but that's not reality. If you follow the lives of most people on the show, you'll learn that they put the weight back on again.

Thankfully God always provides the template for how we are to live life, and it includes His blueprint for victory over strongholds. Like working out in the gym, we don't see the results right away. It takes time, patience, and a whole lot of sweat equity.

As the Israelites marched out of Egypt through the Red Sea and into the wilderness, God promised He would be with them through the entire journey.

He also promised He would help them have victory over all of their enemies and was very specific on how He would help them. God says, *"I will drive them out little by little until you have increased enough to take possession of the land"* (Exodus 23:30). Why would an all-powerful God take His time to act?

Because God created us, He has the ultimate understanding of human psychology and the process of change.

God's plan to drive out their enemies little by little was also about developing persistence, patience, strategy, and submission. These skills would be essential not only for conquering the land, but also for the Israelites' long-term success and growth as a nation.

God is not just interested in providing quick fixes or instant solutions. He values character development and maturity. By allowing the Israelites to face challenges and adversaries over time, God was giving them the opportunity to build resilience, faith, and character. This process of gradual victory was a means of shaping them into people who could trust and rely on Him in all circumstances.

God's desire was for the Israelites to learn valuable lessons along with receiving His blessings. Similarly, in your health journey, the process of gradual change teaches you discipline, self-control, and the importance of perseverance. These are the fruits of the Spirit that God is cultivating in you.

God's approach was strategic for long-term success. Instant victory might have provided temporary relief, but it might not have prepared the Israelites for the responsibilities and challenges of possessing and managing the Promised Land. What about you? How many times have you gained and lost the same amount of weight without ever gaining any real traction? God is concerned with your long-term victory over your strongholds, not your temporal happiness.

Throughout their journey, the Israelites had to trust in God's guidance and provision. Gradual victory reinforced their dependence on Him and their need to seek His guidance and strength. This trust and reliance on God were essential components of their journey and eventual success.

In the same way, the principles applied by God in guiding the Israelites can be relevant to your health goals. By taking gradual steps towards your health goals, you will reap a harvest if you do not give up (Galatians 6:9). God's approach emphasizes that it's not just about reaching the destination but about the journey and the growth that occurs along the way.

In our *Weight Loss, God's Way* programs, we often present an image that serves as a powerful metaphor for the journey of releasing weight. This imagery is designed to provide women with a clear and honest perspective on what their weight release journey truly entails.

Many individuals initially envision this journey as a smooth, straight line, where each passing week effortlessly sheds pounds with minimal effort. However, as they soon come to realize, this idealized perception rarely aligns with their actual experience. In reality, their journey is more akin to a path filled with hills and valleys, each presenting unique challenges and opportunities for growth.

These hills represent the hurdles we all encounter along the way—such as navigating the temptations of holidays, the disruptions of vacations, moments of wavering willpower, and unexpected setbacks like injuries or health issues. They are the instances that can make the path seem steep and challenging.

> **It's not about constant perfection or uninterrupted progress; it's about resilience, determination, and faith. It's about learning to navigate the ups and downs with grace and perseverance, understanding that these very challenges are an integral part of the transformation process.**

Yet it's by overcoming these hills and valleys that women discover the truth about their weight release journey. It's not about constant perfection or uninterrupted progress, it's about resilience, determination, and faith. It's about learning to navigate the ups and downs with grace and perseverance, understanding that these very challenges are an integral part of the transformation process. It's about continually showing up for yourself each day and surrendering the journey to God.

The image we share serves as a reminder that, while the journey may have its moments of difficulty and uncertainty, it is in embracing these challenges that women find their true strength. It's about navigating the hills and valleys, learning and growing along the way, and ultimately emerging on the other side, transformed not only in body but also in spirit. It's a journey where setbacks are not failures but stepping stones toward a healthier, more vibrant, and God-empowered life.

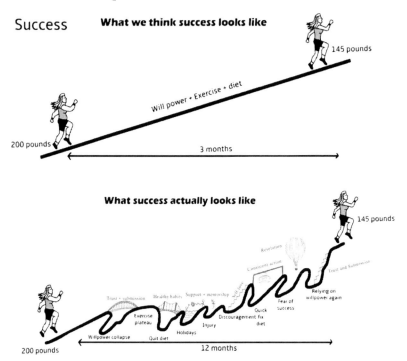

Download a printable version at: breakthroughmethodbonus.com

Principle 7 Summary

Reflect on these key points:

- Set S.M.A.R.T goals for success.
- Understand the gradual process, little by little.
- Emphasize long-term success over temporary happiness.

Principle #8: Develop Emotional Resilience

Managing Your Emotions

Do you ever feel like your emotions have a stronghold over you? Perhaps you've noticed that food has become your default response to various emotions you experience.

- You're angry—you eat.

- You're tired—you eat.

- You're frustrated—you eat.

- You're happy—you eat.

It's as if your emotions dictate the course of your day, influencing your food choices, your interactions with others, your outfit selection, and even your work productivity. Unfortunately, our emotions can sometimes surprise us and sabotage our best intentions. This is where principle #8, managing your emotions, comes into play.

Emotional eating is a complex and deeply ingrained behavior that many of us struggle with. It's the act of eating in response to our emotions rather than true physical hunger. We use food as a coping mechanism, a source of comfort, or a way to numb emotional pain. These eating patterns often become automatic and subconscious, making them challenging to break free from. So just how do we overcome emotional eating if it's subconscious? Most of us focus on the symptom. We try to stop ourselves from emotional eating but, as you can probably attest, that seldom works. Your assignment will be to dismantle your current habit of reacting to your emotions by eating. You will get skilled at feeling your feelings, instead feeding them with food.

To understand the role of emotions and how they impact your weight, I think it's worth understanding the importance of our emotions in the context of our original design.

In Genesis 2:7, the Bible says: "Then the LORD God formed man (Adam) from the dust of the ground and breathed into his nostrils the breath of life, and the man became a living being." Here we see God creating Adam in His image as a three-part being: spirit, soul, and body. God created man from the "dust from the ground," which refers to his body; "breathed into his nostrils the breath of life" refers to man's spirit; and when God's Spirit infused with the physical body, man's soul was created. It is this tripartite nature that empowers us to navigate the intricate world of emotions and discover and develop emotional resilience. In addition to our emotions, our mind, will, consciousness, and feelings also find their home in the place we refer to as our soul.

Your emotions are a complex mix of feelings like joy, sorrow, anger, fear, and love. It's where your deepest passions and vulnerabilities reside, making it a potent and often overpowering force in your life. Your emotions possess the power to elevate you to great heights, filling your heart with the warmth of love, the thrill of joy, and the passion of purpose. Yet they can also plunge you into the depths of despair, igniting the flames of anger, the chill of fear, and the weight of sadness. This dance of emotions, while complicated, is an integral part of God's creative design for us. Emotions color your world, giving it depth and meaning. However, for many of us, emotions have not always been friends; they've often been perceived as adversaries, wielding a powerful influence on our relationship with food. You may relate to the times when emotions have seemingly hijacked your choices, leading you down a path where food became your refuge, a crutch, or a distraction from emotional turmoil.

The connection between emotions and eating isn't just a random occurrence—it's deeply rooted in our human nature. Emotions play a significant role in our decisions about what, when, and how much we eat. In moments of celebration, we indulge in comfort foods to enhance our joy. When stress and anxiety creep in, we may find solace in a bag of chips or a bowl of ice cream. Emotions often become the compass that guides our food choices, directing us toward foods that offer a temporary respite from emotional turmoil.

While it's natural for emotions to influence your eating habits, it becomes problematic when they dictate the course of your life; when food becomes the go-to solution for every emotional twist and turn. You may find yourself caught in the cycle of emotional eating, where food acts as a buffer between you and your emotions.

As you pursue the path to emotional resilience, you will be confronted with the opportunity to transform your relationship with your emotions. Rather than being governed by them, you can learn to navigate this realm using emotions as guides to lead you toward more nutritious food, as well as, life choices.

Your journey into emotional resilience is about embracing the full spectrum of your emotions and surrendering them to God, allowing Him to meet all your emotional needs. It's about recognizing that emotions are not to be feared, suppressed, or buried beneath layers of comfort food. Instead they are to be apprehended, acknowledged, and aligned with God. Emotions serve as beacons illuminating the path to greater self-awareness and healing. By exploring your emotions, you will gain a deeper insight into your true desires, needs, and triggers.

> **Your journey into emotional resilience is about embracing the full spectrum of your emotions and surrendering them to God, allowing Him to meet all your emotional needs.**

In the pages that follow, we'll voyage into the heart of emotional resilience. We'll unpack the intricacies of our emotions, seeking to understand their role in our relationship with food. We'll discover how to feel our feelings without feeding them with food, rewriting the narratives that have long governed our emotional responses.

This chapter isn't about merely stopping yourself from eating; it's about cultivating emotional intelligence, uprooting old beliefs, and developing healthier ways of coping with life's challenges. Together, we'll navigate the path to emotional resilience, recognizing that emotions are not our adversaries but our allies on our journey toward vibrant health.

God and Emotions

In the beginning, when God created you, He gave you a range of emotions as part of His intricate design. These emotions help you navigate life's complexities and connect with both God and others in deep and intimate ways.

However, due to the fallen nature of the world, emotions can become misaligned and dysregulated. In other words, they may not function as they were meant to. Instead of being balanced and appropriately responsive, they can become imbalanced and erratic. Instead of using them as tools for understanding, connection, and growth, we often allow our emotions to control us. This deviation from our intended purpose is a consequence of the brokenness that permeates our human experience.

In Genesis 1:26, we are reminded of our divine calling to have dominion over everything, including our emotions. It's a reminder that we were created to be stewards not only of the physical world but also of our inner world, which includes our thoughts and emotions. Just as we are called to cultivate and care for the Earth, we are also called to cultivate and care for our emotional landscape.

Yet in our broken state, we often find ourselves in a struggle for dominion over our own emotions. They can become unruly masters, dictating our actions and decisions without our conscious consent. This imbalance is what leads to our destructive emotional eating patterns.

Just as a skilled gardener tends to the soil by planting seeds of joy, gratitude, and self-compassion, we too can cultivate a fertile emotional landscape within ourselves. It starts with acknowledging that we have been given the authority to rule over our emotions, to guide them towards health and wholeness.

In the pages that follow, you will learn how to develop emotional mastery, seeking to align your emotions with God's intended purpose for your life. It's a path towards greater self-awareness, resilience, and ultimately, freedom from the chains of emotional eating.

When you grasp the divine purpose behind your emotions, you will realize that they are intended to point you toward God's truth and His presence. Emotions can act as indicators, revealing areas in your life that require attention, healing, or alignment with God's will. By reframing your response to emotions, you can bring them under God's authority, use them as a tool to inform your choices and decisions, and seek God's guidance to understand the root causes of our feelings.

Emotions as Indicators

> *"Be angry and do not sin; do not let the sun go down on your anger, and give no opportunity to the devil." (Eph. 4:26-27 ESV)*

In Ephesians 4, the Apostle Paul teaches us this wisdom on how to effectively navigate life's various stresses, whether they originate externally from conflicts with others or internally from our emotional turmoil. Although his words were initially directed at interpersonal conflicts, their application extends to managing our inner emotional struggles, too.

Paul acknowledges the reality of experiencing emotions, including anger and other intense feelings. He doesn't condemn the presence of these emotions but rather provides guidance on how to handle them in a Godly and constructive manner. This perspective teaches us that emotions are a natural part of the human experience.

However, the key message in Paul's teachings is the importance of addressing and managing our emotions instead of allowing them to control our actions. Unresolved emotional issues can create openings for negative influences to operate in our lives, which is why Paul emphasizes the need to deal with these emotions appropriately.

Paul's counsel encourages us to reflect on our emotional responses and evaluate whether they align with our Christian values and principles. He underscores the significance of processing emotions in ways that are consistent with our faith and belief in God's guidance. When we confront our emotional struggles and seek Godly resolutions we create a space for God's wisdom, healing, and transformation to work in our lives.

> *"Tremble [with anger or fear], and do not sin; Meditate in your heart upon your bed and be still [reflect on your sin and repent of your rebellion]." (Psalms 4:4 AMP)*

Similarly, the psalmist's advice in Psalms 4:4 urges us to examine our hearts and remain silent in moments of anger. This practice encourages self-reflection and restraint, enabling us to gain insight into the root causes of our emotions. Instead of reacting impulsively to anger or other intense feelings, we are encouraged to turn inward, seeking understanding and spiritual alignment.

Both Paul's teachings in Ephesians 4 and the psalmist's guidance in Psalms 4:4 emphasize the importance of using our emotions as a tool for self-awareness and spiritual growth. Emotions can serve as indicators of areas in our lives that require attention, healing, or alignment with God's will. You can seek comfort and guidance from God rather than turning to food as a substitute. This shift will not only transform your relationship with food but also deepen your spiritual connection as you learn to experience emotional well-being in the way God intended.

The Science of Emotion

Let's break down this new awareness of seeing your emotions as indicators or tools for self-awareness and help you to overcome emotional eating.

Picture your emotions as an oversensitive smoke detector within you. Just as a smoke detector can respond to even the slightest hint of smoke, our emotions can react intensely to various situations—even those that might not necessarily pose a real threat.

When your emotions are on high alert due to stress, anxiety, sadness or other triggers, they send signals to your brain that something is amiss. This heightened emotional state can create a sense of discomfort or unease, much like a smoke detector blaring its alarm. And just as we instinctively seek to silence the blaring alarm, we often seek ways to soothe our heightened emotions.

Emotional eating can become a way to temporarily quiet the alarms of your emotions. When you're feeling overwhelmed or distressed, your brain craves relief. Food—especially comfort foods that are often high in sugar, fat, and salt—can provide that temporary sense of comfort and distraction. Just as you might fan away smoke to make the detector stop, you turn to food to calm your emotional alarms.

However, just like fanning to silence a smoke detector doesn't address the underlying issue of a potential fire, emotional eating doesn't address the root causes of your emotional distress. It merely provides a momentary escape but the distress remains, causing the need for more escape. Over time this pattern can become a habit, leading to a cycle where you consistently turn to food as a way to cope with emotions.

To break this cycle, you need to address the emotional triggers themselves rather than just the symptoms. Just as we would address the cause of smoke in the air, you must explore what is causing your emotional distress.

In my case, as I learned to pause and pay attention to what I was truly craving, the Lord revealed to me that at the root was a perpetual feeling of disappointment. I believed that I was a disappointment and I would always be regardless of what I did. As I surrendered this feeling to God and allowed Him to satisfy my unmet core needs, I no longer needed to feed my feelings of disappointment, praise God.

By recognizing that emotional eating is a response to our emotions' alarms, we can begin to develop healthier ways of managing our feelings. Instead of reaching for food, we can turn to strategies that address the root causes of our distress and provide lasting relief. As we learn to manage our emotions in a balanced and mindful way, we can break free from the cycle of emotional eating and find healthier avenues for emotional well-being.

Applying the 3-Step Reset to the Apple Test

Let's go to our 3-Step Reset to help you begin this process of developing your emotional resiliency. We introduced the invaluable tool in Principle 4 as we discussed stress management. You learned how to pause and calm your nervous system by developing an awareness of what's pulling you out of alignment and then surrendering it to God.

In this chapter you will combine the reset with another powerful tool called the "Apple Test". It's a concept and practice used in some counseling and therapy settings to help individuals assess their cravings and eating habits. It's a simple tool you can use to distinguish between real hunger and emotional hunger. That means, before reaching for any food, asking yourself if you would be willing to eat an apple, vegetable, or other healthy snack at that moment.

If the thought of eating an apple seems unappealing or unsatisfying, it might be a sign that your hunger is more emotional than physical. Emotional hunger often craves specific types of foods, like sweets, chips, or fast food. Whereas if you're genuinely hungry, the idea of eating an apple should feel reasonable and even appealing. Your body needs nourishment, and you'd be willing to consume something wholesome to satisfy that hunger.

Now let's combine these two tools.

The 3-Step Reset is going to serve two purposes when it comes to emotional eating.

It's going to help you to tune in and pay attention to whether you're truly hungry or if your cravings are emotional.

Let's begin. Let's say you're craving something to eat.

Step 1: Pause. When you feel the urge to eat, especially if it's not mealtime, take a moment to pause. In the case of emotional eating you're going to insert "The Apple Test" into your pause.

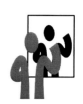

If you find yourself in the pause of the 3-Step Reset and realize that you're not craving an apple but rather your favorite indulgent treat, it's an important moment to dig deeper into your emotions.

During this pause, turn inward and explore your true feelings. Your usual response might involve using food to comfort your emotions. However, emotions are meant to be experienced, offering you deeper insights into your soul. Your goal is to feel them and bring them into union with your Heavenly Father by reflecting on the following questions:

1. **What emotion am I experiencing?** Try to pinpoint the emotion that's bubbling up within you. Is it sadness, frustration, anxiety, loneliness, or perhaps a combination of these? Identifying the core emotion is a crucial step in addressing the root cause of your cravings.

2. **What triggered this emotion?** Consider the circumstances or events that might have triggered this emotion. Did you have a disagreement with someone? Did a situation not unfold as you expected or hoped? Understanding the trigger can provide valuable insights into why you're turning to food for comfort.

3. **Am I using food to numb or avoid feelings?** Pay attention and notice if you're using food as a coping mechanism to numb or distract yourself from uncomfortable emotions. This self-awareness is the first step toward breaking free from emotional eating patterns.

Step 2: Pray. Once you've paused and reflected on your emotions and cravings, the next step in the 3-Step Reset is to pray.

There are a variety of ways to incorporate prayer into your journey of overcoming emotional eating:

1. **Seek God's presence.** Begin by acknowledging God's presence in your life. Recognize that He is with you in every situation, including this one. Take a moment to center yourself and remember that you are not alone. Acknowledge His presence and surrender everything to Him.

2. **Express your emotions.** Be honest with God about what you're feeling. Share your emotions, fears, frustrations, and even your cravings with Him. Pour out your heart in prayer, knowing that God is a compassionate listener who understands your innermost thoughts and feelings.

3. **Ask for help.** Pray for strength and wisdom to overcome emotional eating. Request God's guidance in discerning the root causes of your cravings and emotions. Ask Him to empower you to make healthier choices and resist the urge to use food as a coping mechanism.

4. **Declare God's promises.** Speak God's promises and affirmations

over yourself. Remind yourself of scriptures that emphasize His love, grace, and strength. For example, you can declare Philippians 4:13: "I can do all things through Christ who strengthens me" as a source of empowerment.

5. **Listen in silence.** After you've poured out your heart, take a moment to listen in silence. Be receptive to any guidance or insights that God may provide during this time of prayer. His still, small voice can illuminate your path forward. It's also helpful to journal what He's saying to you.

6. **Express gratitude.** Conclude your prayer with a heart of gratitude. Thank God for His presence, love, and willingness to walk with you on this journey. Express faith in His ability to bring transformation into your life.

Depending on your circumstance or situation, your prayer might come in the form of a confession or declaration. It might not always be convenient or practical to go to God's Word, but we can always make these confessions and declarations in our head. Here's some we use in the Weight Loss, God's Way program:

- "God is in control."
- "What's important is what God thinks of me."
- "My assignment is to please God, not man."
- "I am loved lavishly by God."
- "I deserve to take care of myself."
- "I am made in the image of God."
- "God will fight for me."

Declarations

These declarations are grounded in Scripture, and you can use them to renew your mind when you find yourself out of alignment with God's best for you. This is a short prayer to God that you can repeat throughout the day as many times as you need. Keep one (or more) on your phone or somewhere that you can quickly access it when you need it. Here are a few examples:

- "Thank You, God, that You are healing/helping/strengthening/working on me according to Your perfect schedule."

- "Your grace is sufficient."

- "Lord, I choose to stand in Your truth and not worry about what's happening around me. You are in control, and that's all that matters."

- "Thank You, God, for being my source of comfort and strength. When my emotions pull me toward food, I choose to turn to You for solace. Your presence fills the void that emotional eating cannot. I trust in Your perfect plan for my emotional well-being."

- "I thank You, God, for creating me in Your image, with a spirit, soul, and body. I turn to You for strength and guidance. You've designed me for a deeper connection with You, and I embrace my value and worth in Your eyes."

- "Lord, I thank You that my greatest desire is to know You intimately and earnestly. I see myself as valuable and beautiful just as You see me."

Feel free to use these declarations as a tool to renew your mind and find strength in God's grace when faced with unruly emotions.

Scriptures/Confessions

These are perfect to use when you're journaling or just need to be strengthened by God's Word.

- I am confident that God will perfect the work He has begun in me (Phil. 1:6).

- I have not been given a spirit of fear, but of power, love, and self-discipline (2 Tim. 1:7).

- I am given God's glorious grace lavishly and without restriction (Eph. 1:5,8).

- I am assured all things work together for good (Rom. 8:28).

- I have peace (Eph. 2:14).

- I am chosen and dearly loved by God (1 Thes. 1:4).

- I am created in the image of God (2 Cor. 4:4).

- I am not helpless (Phil. 4:13).

- I am blessed in the heavenly realms with every spiritual blessing (Eph. 1:3).

- I can be kind and compassionate to others (Eph. 4:32).

- I am set free (Rom. 8:2; Jn. 8:32).

- My heart and mind are protected with God's peace (Phil. 4:7).

- I possess the mind of Christ (1 Cor. 2:16).

Step 3. Active Practice. After you've paused to reflect, prayed for guidance and strength, the final step is your "Active Practice". Remember, your Active Practice involves taking specific actions or gestures in response to your thoughts and emotions. This can be done in conjunction with Step 2. For example, if your declaration is "I am strong and resilient", your Active Practice might involve physically flexing your muscles.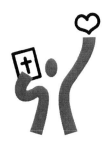

Commit to performing your chosen Active Practice consistently throughout the day whenever this emotion arises. Repetition is key to rewiring your brain and creating new and healthier habits.

When you engage in your Active Practice, do it mindfully. Focus on the intention behind the action and its connection to your declarations. Visualize yourself breaking free from the negative thought patterns and cravings as you perform the practice.

As you practice this 3-Step Reset regularly, you'll develop a greater capacity to address the root causes of emotional eating, ultimately leading to greater healing and transformation on your weight-release journey.

By using this simple tool you'll develop self-awareness, emotional understanding, and spiritual growth. It's about replacing old habits with new, faith-based practices that support both your well-being and your connection with God's truth.

A final caveat in this chapter: Don't forget to give yourself lots of grace, which is crucial on your journey to managing your emotions. The goal is not to try to stop yourself from feeling, and don't beat up on yourself when you don't practice the 3-Step Reset. Recognize that this process can be challenging, and there may be times when you struggle to turn to God or when you pray you still find yourself succumbing to emotional eating. In these moments, remember the concept of grace and offer yourself the same compassion and understanding that God extends to you.

Here's why grace is so important:

1. **Recognizes Your Humanity.** Emotional eating, like many other challenges in life, is a part of your human experience. We all have moments of weakness and vulnerability. By acknowledging your humanity, you avoid self-condemnation, guilt and shame, which can often exacerbate emotional eating patterns. Instead, you cultivate self-compassion.

2. **God's Unconditional Love.** God's love for you is unwavering and unconditional. He doesn't withhold His love or grace when you stumble. Instead, He offers His grace as a source of strength and encouragement. Knowing that you are unconditionally loved by God can give you the confidence to keep seeking His help, even in the face of setbacks.

3. **Learn and Grow.** Every step of this journey is an opportunity for learning and growth. When you extend grace to yourself, you create an environment conducive to self-improvement. It's through these experiences, even the challenging ones, that you gain insight, build resilience, and develop a deeper connection with God.

4. **Avoids the Shame Spiral.** The shame associated with emotional eating can create a destructive cycle. You eat emotionally, feel guilty, eat more to cope with the guilt, and the cycle continues. Embracing grace helps break this pattern. When you forgive yourself and acknowledge that each day is a new opportunity, you interrupt the shame spiral and allow for healing to take place.

5. **Maintains Your Connection with God.** Emotional eating can sometimes lead to feelings of distance from God. You might feel unworthy

or disconnected. Embracing grace allows you to maintain your connection with God, understanding that He is always there, ready to offer guidance and support when you turn to Him.

6. **Builds Trust.** I'm going to keep reminding you to trust in the process and in your relationship with God. Grace plays a vital role in building and strengthening that trust. As you experience God's grace, you learn to trust that His love and support are unwavering, regardless of your challenges.

Grace is the gentle, loving hand that guides you through the journey of managing emotional eating. It reminds you that you are human, that God's love is unconditional, and that each moment is an opportunity for growth and connection. Embrace grace as your companion on this path, and let it be a source of comfort, strength, and encouragement when you face the inevitable bumps along the way.

Principle 8 Summary

Reflect on these key points:

- Emotional resilience is developed as you understand what's driving your emotions.

- Reframe emotions to a helpful tool like a smoke detector, signaling potential issues.

- Emotions are part of God's design for navigating life, but they can be misused. Our responsibility is to have dominion over our emotions, as mentioned in Genesis 1:26, by practicing the 3-Step Reset

---

Principle #9: Develop a System

Master Your Routine

As I write this chapter, I find myself ten days into the month, realizing that I haven't even begun to check off my monthly habit checklist, and I'm a couple of months behind on my productivity planner. It's just a simple check mark on a piece of paper, I tell myself, so what's been keeping me from doing it? That's the thing about establishing new habits. They're easy to do, but they're also easy not to do. When I consistently track the habits I want to master, it simplifies my life and helps me keep my priorities in check. However, when I don't do it, I can feel the difference. Each day, I keep telling myself, "I'll start tomorrow". Yet here we are, ten days into the month, and each "tomorrow" becomes "today", which quickly turns into "yesterday".

It's the tools like my monthly habit checklist (download at breakthrough-methodbonus.com) and my productivity planner that have helped me master many of my habits, allowing me to achieve high levels of productivity and energy each day. My morning routine, workout routine, eating routine, work routine, and sleep routine are pretty dialed in, although I continue to work on mastering them. The goal is simplicity. How can I put the day-to-day routine tasks on autopilot so I can set it and forget it? How can I ensure that the little but important things like flossing my teeth, taking my vitamins, staying hydrated, checking in with family, and journaling all get done each day?

It's the everyday, consistent habits that hold the key to your most significant breakthroughs. These daily rhythms are the small hinges that effortlessly swing open the doors to lasting change. However, despite our best intentions, many of us struggle to establish these essential routines for our health. Life is busier than ever, with constant distractions vying for our attention. We find ourselves pulled in many directions, and all too often our priorities get reordered by a constant barrage of images, subtly and not-so-subtly influencing our choices. I can't count the number of times I've logged onto my computer for a work task, only to find myself still caught up in the vortex of Instagram videos an hour later. I've ended up with items in my cart that I felt I couldn't live without, even though I didn't know I needed them. Worst of all, I can't even remember what I initially went on the computer for! Companies spend millions of dollars hijacking our attention, and we are no match for their tactics. That's why we need a system.

Without a reliable system in place, we often end up majoring in the minors or succumbing to the path of least resistance when faced with choices and tasks. We gravitate toward the easiest or most familiar options, even when they may not serve our best interests. It's time to develop a system that will guide us in making better choices, reclaiming our priorities, and simplifying our lives.

That's why Principle #9 is "Develop a System."

Without a well-defined system in place, you might find yourself moving through your day making choices based on convenience rather than what's healthiest for you. It's much easier to grab fast food on the way home from work than to prepare a nutritious meal from scratch. It's simpler to skip the gym and watch TV instead of following a regular exercise routine. It's more comfortable to stay up late scrolling through social media than to prioritize a good night's sleep.

The path of least resistance is the path that doesn't require much effort or discomfort. It's the path that feels immediately gratifying, but it rarely leads to long-term benefits. When it comes to your health, it's probably the path of least resistance that has brought you to your current state of health.

But with a system, you can change this. A system, in this context, refers to a set of interconnected actions, routines, and habits that work together to support your goals. Without a system you're left with a series of inconsistent actions, making it difficult to maintain consistency and make meaningful progress. It will often feel like you're taking one step forward and two steps back. Can you relate?

In this chapter, you'll explore how to build such systems for your health and life. Particular emphasis will be placed on your morning and evening routines, as they serve as the foundational bookends framing your success. You'll learn how to design routines and habits that become the new path of least resistance, making it easier for you to consistently prioritize your health. By doing so, you'll empower yourself to make choices that align with your goals so that you can achieve your healthy weight without feeling like you're always starting over or like you're aiming at a moving target.

Why You Need a S.Y.S.T.E.M.

Some time ago, I came across a valuable acronym that resonated deeply with me, and I'd like to share it with you. S.Y.S.T.E.M., which stands for 'Save Yourself Stress, Time, Energy, and Money,' perfectly summarizes the impact it can have on your weight-releasing journey.

Save Yourself Stress

Planning and Preparation: Establishing routines and systems in your weight-releasing journey can significantly reduce stress. When you plan meals, workouts, and other health-related activities in advance as part of your routine, you minimize the stress of making last-minute decisions or facing uncertainty about your daily choices.

Save Yourself Time

Efficient Time Management: Structured routines help you manage your time efficiently. Just think of how much time you've wasted procrastinating or spending time trying to figure out what to eat.

Save Yourself Energy

Conservation of Mental Energy: Routines conserve mental energy by eliminating the need to constantly think about what to do next, what to eat, what to wear, and what to cook. When your weight-releasing activities are part of your daily system, you expend less mental effort on decision-making and planning. Then there's all the emotional energy wasted on all the guilt, shame, worry, and anxiety associated with trying to lose weight.

Save Yourself Money

Meal Planning: By planning your meals and snacks, you can make cost-effective choices, avoid unnecessary dining out or eating in, and reduce food waste, which ultimately saves you money. Let's not even talk about all the money that's been spent on diet programs that had little to no impact.

Having a system not only supports your physical health and weight release goals but also contributes to overall well-being by reducing stress and optimizing resource management.

Routines and Habit Stacking

In his book *Atomic Habits*, James Clear emphasizes the power of small, incremental changes in building lasting habits. Habit stacking is one of the techniques he highlights to make these changes more manageable and effective.

Habit stacking is a powerful technique that helps you establish new habits by integrating them into your existing routines. It's a practical approach to building a series of habits that flow seamlessly from one to the next, making it easier to incorporate new behaviors into your daily life.

Here's how habit stacking works:

Identify Your Current Routine. Start by listing your existing daily routines. These are the actions and habits you consistently perform, such as your morning routine, evening routine, or work-related tasks.

Define Your New Habit. Clearly specify the new habit you want to incorporate into your routine. Whether it's related to nutritious eating, exercise, sleep, or stress management, be precise about what you want to achieve.

Find a Trigger. Choose a habit from your current routine that can serve as a trigger for the new habit. This should be a task you already do regularly and consistently.

Establish a Clear Connection. Clearly connect the new habit to the trigger habit. You should be able to say, "After [current habit], I will [new habit]." This connection makes it easier to remember and implement.

Repeat and Refine. Practice this habit stacking consistently. Over time, it becomes an automatic part of your routine. If you encounter difficulties, adjust the timing, or choose a different trigger habit until the new habit becomes established.

Let's look at how we can incorporate habit stacking to help you establish consistent routines with your Core Four habits.

1. Healthy Eating

    Morning Routine: If your morning routine includes a cup of tea or coffee, you can habit stack by taking your vitamins with your coffee. This may even lead to stacking on a new habit of drinking some water in the future.

    Meal Preparation: When you prepare meals or snacks, you can habit stack by incorporating time to plan out your next meal, take your vitamins, or even drinking a cup of water.

2. Physical Activity

    Morning Routine: After your morning prayer time, you can habit stack by adding a brief stretching session. After your quiet time, spend a few minutes doing simple stretches to wake up your body and pre-pare it for the day. Personally, I do a two - minute wall squat while brushing my teeth.

    Evening Routine: Before bedtime, as you put on your night clothes, include a habit of setting out your workout clothes for the next day. This prepares you mentally and reduces the friction of exercise prepa-ration in the morning.

3. Adequate Sleep

    Evening Routine: When winding down for sleep, you can habit stack by adding a relaxation technique like deep breathing or gentle stretch-es. Incorporating these practices into your evening routine can signal to your body that it's time to rest.

4. Effective Stress Management

Morning Routine: During your prayer time, create a habit of surrendering everything you will eat to God.

Work Routine: While at work or during your daily tasks, stack stress management by taking a couple of deep breaths before answering the phone, do a few stretches before or after getting up to use the restroom, or even perform your Active Practice. These small interludes can help you manage stress and stay focused.

As you link these new habits to the routines you already follow, you create a structure that promotes consistency and success in maintaining your health goals.

Now let's go into more detail so that you can plan out your morning routine.

Establishing a Morning Routine

Routines help you form habits, and habits simplify life because when something becomes habituated, you don't have to think about it. You can set it and forget it.

Establishing a morning routine sets a positive tone for your day. It allows you to surrender your agenda to God and seek His guidance, inspiration, and the strength you need for the day ahead.

A morning routine that includes prayer, some exercise, planning, and hydrating will help reduce your stress levels and feelings of being overwhelmed. Lower stress levels prevent emotional eating throughout the day.

Morning exercise can jumpstart your metabolism, boost energy levels, and set the stage for healthier choices throughout the day. It sets you up for success.

Having a morning routine can give you the foresight you need to plan out your day and help you manage your time efficiently. By allocating specific slots for self-care, exercise, and meal preparation, you optimize your schedule and make room for activities that support your weight-release goals.

With a morning routine, you won't be caught off guard later in the day about what you should eat, and you're more likely to pay attention to what you eat and how you eat it.

Here are the steps to create a morning routine:

1. **Determine Your Wake-Up Time.** The key to a successful morning routine starts with waking up at a consistent time each day. Your wake-up time should be tailored to your personal sleep needs, ensuring you get the recommended 7-9 hours of restful sleep each night. A consistent wake-up time helps regulate your internal body clock, making it easier to rise and shine.

2. **Allocate Morning Time.** Once you've determined your wake-up time, calculate the amount of time you have available each morning based on when you need to start your day. This allows you to plan your activities effectively.

3. **Prioritize Essential Activities.** Your morning routine should ideally encompass key activities that set a positive tone for your day. These essentials may include:

   • Worship or Reflection: Begin your day by connecting with God or the Word or engaging in a moment of mindfulness and gratitude.

   • Hydration: Kickstart your metabolism and rehydrate your body with a glass of water upon waking. If you're planning to exercise, consider drinking more.

   • Exercise: The duration of an exercise routine can vary based on your preferences and available time. It might range from a quick stretching session to a full workout.

   • Breakfast: Allow yourself ample time to mindfully enjoy a nutritious breakfast. Eating slowly and savoring your meal can lead to better digestion and overall satisfaction.

   • Day Planning: Invest a few minutes to review your schedule, set priorities, and organize tasks for the day ahead.

   • Meal Prep: While it's ideal to prepare meals the night before, allocate time in your morning routine, if needed, to ensure you're not tempted by unhealthy fast food options throughout the day.

- Habit Stacking: Incorporate new habits into existing routines. For example, you can link your morning prayer or meditation with your hydration habit, reinforcing both practices.

4. **Morning Prayer or Meditation.** Dedicate a portion of your morning routine to fellowshipping with God. Commit to surrendering everything and everyone to Him and make restoring union with God your goal.

5. **Start Slowly.** If you're new to morning routines, don't feel compelled to tackle each activity with full intensity right away. You can start with shorter durations for each task, gradually extending the time as you become more comfortable and the routine becomes more ingrained.

6. **Stay Consistent.** Consistency in your wake-up time and the order of your activities is essential. A consistent routine will help your body adapt to this new schedule, making it feel natural and effortless.

7. **Adjust as Needed.** Be flexible and willing to adjust the time allocated to each activity based on your daily schedule. If you have a particularly busy morning you might need to shorten some activities temporarily, but always aim to maintain the core components of your routine.

By carefully considering and implementing these points, you can create a morning routine that promotes a healthy start to your day, ensuring you're well-prepared to live out the Core Four principles consistently.

Here is a sample routine:

Sample Morning Routine	
Time	**Activity**
6:00 AM	Wake up
6:10 AM	Prayer
6:35 AM	Hydrate (drink water)
6:40 AM	Light Stretching
6:50 AM	Breakfast (nutritious)

7:15 AM	Make lunch
7:30 AM	Review daily tasks
8:00 AM	Exercise (e.g., jog, pilates)
8:30 AM	Shower and get dressed
9:00 AM	Start work

Establishing an Evening Routine

In order to establish a morning routine, it really starts the night before with your evening routine because the time you go to bed will determine the time you wake up.

Having a consistent evening routine provides closure for your day, allowing you to wind down and prepare for the upcoming day. It is one of the keys to successful weight releasing.

How to Create an Evening Routine

- **Determine Your Sleep Time.** Begin by identifying what time you need to wake up to get 7-9 hours of sleep. For example, if you need to wake up at 6:00 AM, you should aim to be in bed between 9:00 PM and 11:00 PM.

- **Calculate Backwards.** Once you have your wake-up time, work backward to determine when your evening routine should start. Consider how much time you typically need to wind down and complete your routine activities. I suggest you start your routine when you get home from work or whatever time you designate as the end of your work day.

- **Allocate Time for Dinner.** Ideally, plan to have dinner at least three hours before your bedtime. This allows your body time to digest food properly before sleep. If dinner preparation is part of your routine, allocate time for meal prep as well. Whenever possible, meal prep on the weekends to maximize your weekday time in the kitchen. Allocate at least 15-20 minutes to enjoy your dinner mindfully

127

without rushing. Chew your food slowly, enjoying every bit. Avoid eating in front of the TV or a screen. Instead, focus on savoring your meal and listening to your body's hunger cues.

- **Minimize Distractions.** Minimize your TV watching time and other distractions that will quickly suck up your time. Plan your TV watching time and stick to it.

- **Relaxation Activities.** Incorporate relaxation techniques into your evening routine to help you unwind. This could be as soon as you end your workday or after dinner. Activities like reading, gentle stretching, or deep breathing exercises can promote relaxation and reduce stress.

- **Digital Detox.** Set a specific time to disconnect from electronic devices like smartphones, tablets, and computers. The blue light from screens can interfere with your body's natural sleep-wake cycle, making it harder to fall asleep.

- **Personal Care.** Dedicate time for personal care activities such as skincare, brushing your teeth, and preparing for the next day. This can take around 15-30 minutes, depending on your routine.

- **Evening Prayer or Reflection.** End your day with God. Recap the day and renew your mind in any areas that you felt could use a redo. Do this in your mind by reflecting on how you would do it differently the next time.

- **Prep for the Next Day.** Spend a few minutes organizing your belongings, setting out clothes for the next day, and making a to-do list. This helps reduce morning stress and allows for a smoother start to your day.

- **Time for Rest.** As you approach your bedtime, ensure you have enough time for a full night's sleep. Avoid activities that may stimulate your mind or increase stress levels, such as intense work tasks or engaging in emotionally charged conversations. Avoid watching the news!

- **Consistency.** Try to stick to the same bedtime and evening routine consistently, even on weekends. Consistency helps regulate your body's internal clock and improves sleep quality.

- **Adjust as Needed.** Be flexible with your routine. Life events or changes in your schedule may require adjustments to your evening routine. The key is to maintain the overall structure to support restful sleep and holistic health.

Sample Evening Routine	
Time	**Activity**
6:00 PM	Finish dinner
6:30 PM	Tidy up living space
7:00 PM	Relaxation (read, listen to music)
7:30 PM	Prayer
7:45 PM	Gratitude journaling
8:00 PM	Light stretching
8:15 PM	Prepare for the next day (lay out clothes, pack essentials)
8:30 PM	Wind down (dim lights, limit screen time)
9:00 PM	Bedtime

Repetition is Key

As we said at the outset of this lesson, establishing routines can be difficult because our natural makeup is to take the path of least resistance. This may serve us in some areas of life, but in the area of weight releasing it's not helpful. So, let's look at how we can develop the skills necessary to master our routines and create lasting health habits.

Repetition is vital to developing and maintaining routines because it strengthens the neural connections in your brain. This makes it easier for your brain to initiate and execute the routine in the future. Over time, this neural efficiency makes it feel more natural and less effortful to follow the routine.

Yet too often, when most people set off on a weight releasing journey, they quit when they don't see results. If only they could understand the importance of repetition. The need to keep showing up for yourself day in and day out.

When you go to the gym, you don't expect immediate transformation. It's the consistent, repeated effort over time that builds strength, endurance, and a healthier body. The act of working out becomes a routine, something you do regularly because you understand that it's the repetition that brings about change. In the same way, your daily habits related to health should be repeated consistently to make a significant impact.

Or take the simple habit of brushing your teeth daily. It's a well-practiced routine that most people don't even think twice about. It's a habit formed through the repetition of a simple action. Over time, this repetition leads to better oral health. It's not the grand, once-in-a-lifetime gesture but the consistent, everyday brushing that keeps your teeth in great condition. So whether it's your exercise routine, dietary choices, or any other health-related habits, remember that the power lies in the consistent repetition of these actions. This repetition transforms ordinary actions into life-enhancing routines that contribute to your overall well-being.

Here are some practical tools you can also try to help you establish routines:

Set Alarms or Reminders

Just as you set an alarm to wake up in the morning, you can use alarms or reminders on your phone or clock to prompt you to start your routine activities at the designated times. These reminders act as gentle nudges, helping you stay on track with your daily routines. You can use these reminders to alert you when to drink water, get up and go for a walk, take your vitamins, or any other health habit you want to master.

Routine Tracking Apps

In our digital age, there are apps designed specifically to help you track and manage your daily routines. These apps can be incredibly valuable for motivation and progress monitoring. They often provide visual progress tracking, allowing you to see how consistently you've been following your routines. The awareness of your progress can be a great motivator to maintain consistency. A couple of currently popular apps include Done, Routinist, and Habitica.

Visual Aids and Cues

Sometimes, seeing is believing. Create visual aids and cues to reinforce your routines and goals. For example, if part of your morning routine includes exercise, place your gym bag near the door. This visual cue not only reminds you of your commitment but also makes it more convenient to carry out the action. I always keep a glass of water by my bed to remind me to drink a cup of water as soon as I wake up. Additionally, consider creating vision boards that represent your routines and health goals. I used to think vision boards were kind of corny but I gave it a try and created one. I'm amazed at how it serves as daily reminders of my aspirations and helps keep me focused.

In addition to these tools, using the 3-Step Reset will be powerful again here to help you develop consistent routines.

Here's how you can use the 3-Step Reset to master your morning routine with this change:

Step 1: Pause

Upon waking up, before diving into your morning routine, take a moment to pause and reflect. This pause allows you to surrender your day and your habits to God and assess how you feel physically and emotionally.

As you tune in to your body, you can pay attention to your habits more broadly. Maybe you're tempted to reach for your phone and scroll through social media immediately upon waking. Instead, pause and ask yourself if this habit serves your well-being or if it's driven by a need for distraction or validation.

Step 2: Pray for Guidance and Strength

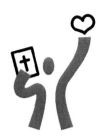

After pausing and reflecting, turn to prayer for guidance and strength. Seek God's wisdom in making choices that align with your values and goals. You might say, "Heavenly Father, grant me the wisdom to make mindful choices this morning and the strength to stay aligned with my intentions."

Step 3: Engage in an Active Practice

Your Active Practice is the power of habit stacking put into action. Every time you perform it, it realigns you with your desires and reminds you to invite God into your journey.

As we conclude this chapter, I want to offer you not just guidance but also encouragement and a sense of hope. The power of your morning and evening routines will make all the difference. They are the perfect bookends to hold your day in place. By embracing the Core Four principles and weaving them into these daily rhythms you're not just creating routines, you're crafting the pathway to lasting transformation as well. These routines are your allies, your guiding lights on the journey to optimal health and weight.

Remember that without routines, we often drift back to the path of least resistance. The gravitational pull of convenience can lead us astray. But by establishing these routines, you are setting yourself up for success. You're creating a life where making healthy choices becomes second nature. It's not about grand, one-time efforts but the consistent, everyday actions that make a profound difference.

So, take heart and approach this with enthusiasm and grace. Your morning and evening routines are the canvas on which you paint the masterpiece of your health journey. Each day, as you follow these routines with intention, you're taking steps closer to being the healthiest and best version of yourself. Keep this vision in mind as you craft your routines, and know that you have the power to make each day a masterpiece, one small, purposeful action at a time.

Principle 9 Summary

Reflect on these key points:

- Recognize that success often stems from making consistent daily habits, not overwhelming changes. Small, repeated actions can lead to significant progress.

- You need a system for success. Habit Stacking is an effective tool to help you add new habits to your existing ones.

- Establishing a consistent morning and evening routine is like two bookends that frame the success of your day.

Principle #10: Schedule Health as a Priority

Put The Big Rocks First

A philosophy professor once stood up before his class with a large empty jar. He filled the jar to the top with large rocks and asked his students if the jar was full.

The students said that 'yes', the jar was full.

He then added small pebbles to the jar, giving the jar an occasional shake so the pebbles could settle among the bigger rocks. Then he asked again, "Is the jar full now?"

Again, the students agreed that the jar was indeed full.

He then poured sand into the jar to fill up any remaining empty space. Once again, the students then agreed that the jar was completely full. Finally, the professor poured water into the jar and watched the water settle among the rocks, pebbles and sand. And he asked, "Is the jar full now?" And once again, the students said that 'yes' the jar was full.

The jar was indeed full at this point so he asked the students the point of this illustration to which someone replied that you could always fit more things into your life if "you really work at it."

"No," countered the professor. "The point is, if you don't put the big rocks in first, you will never be able to fit them in later."

Doesn't it often feel like this is how your day unfolds? You start with good intentions, planning to prioritize activities like prayer, hitting the gym, or enjoying quality time with your spouse or friend. But before you realize it it's 6:00 pm, and you find yourself sitting in the car, in the drive-through lane, wondering where your day disappeared to.

Our daily lives often become overwhelmed with trivial tasks like errands, phone calls, TV, social media, or shopping. To break free from this cycle, it's crucial to shift your approach. Instead of just **prioritizing your schedule, focus on scheduling your priorities.** This means intentionally allocating time for the things that truly matter, such as personal growth, health, quality time with loved ones, or pursuing your life's purpose.

In line with Stephen Covey's wisdom in *The 7 Habits of Highly Effective People*, this shift can be summarized as "Do first things first."

This means that instead of merely deciding what tasks to do when, you should proactively allocate time in your daily schedule for your most important tasks and responsibilities and learn to say 'no' to less important activities. It's a shift from merely thinking about what's important to actually blocking out specific time slots in your schedule for these important tasks or activities.

When You Prioritize Your Schedule

You prioritize the urgent over the important, leading to increased frustration, a constantly growing to-do list, and a lack of peace in your life.

You're driven by external pressures, which can make you feel overwhelmed and result in unwanted consequences like emotional eating.

You put others' needs ahead of your own, which limits your sense of fulfillment and personal growth.

You risk experiencing long-term burnout and feeling disconnected from your deeper sense of purpose by constantly focusing on the urgent.

You may also stray from the best and highest version of who God has called you to be.

When You Schedule Your Priorities

You can deliberately focus on what's truly important, understanding that (other people's) urgent matters can be deferred to a more appropriate time (for you).

You have a sense of accomplishment, as you're actively moving toward your significant, long-term goals.

You experience a greater sense of peace, knowing that your actions align with what you believe God has called you to do, and your choices reflect your faith and values.

As you lie down to rest at night you can sleep with a clear conscience, understanding that you've given your best effort to what matters most to you.

You eliminate the feeling of frustration and the sense of spinning your wheels as you've taken charge of your life.

You experience a deep sense of peace and contentment as your daily actions align with your values and faith.

You notice significant progress toward accomplishing your goals, and your life is moving in a direction that brings fulfillment and purpose.

You have increased confidence in your connection with God, as you're no longer frazzled by the overwhelming demands of countless tasks. Your life is more in tune with God's guidance, and you can more clearly discern His direction.

Sound too good to be true? It is possible!

Understandably, this may feel impossible at the beginning since there may be so many things vying for your attention. But give yourself lots of grace as you practice. It will take a shift in your mindset to begin to think of your priorities this way.

Remember, our tendency is to focus on the urgent, the immediate, the crisis in the moment—the permission forms for school need to be handed in tomorrow; the work deadline that's past due; the dishes are piling up in the sink now; your husband or kids need you to find their socks now; the library books are overdue; the phone call that you've been meaning to return for weeks. All these urgent matters can easily take the place of spending time with God if we allow them. That's why we must continually surrender our days to God and ask Him to order our steps. Here's how you can begin to implement these strategies into your daily life.

How to practically implement this strategy:

1. **Start Your Day with God.** Beginning your day with a spiritual connection to God sets the tone for your entire day. By dedicating these initial moments to God, you acknowledge your dependence on Him and let go of your will.

2. **Prioritize Your Priorities.** By scheduling the most important things into your day before anything else. Begin your day with prayer time, exercise, and quality time with family, placing these essential activities ahead of tasks like laundry, returning calls, checking emails, or watching TV.

3. **Weekly Planning.** Dedicate time every Sunday to schedule your priorities for the week. This intentional planning session allows you to set your intentions and identify what truly matters to you in the upcoming week.

4. **Nightly Routine.** Before you go to bed each night, invest a few minutes in plugging your priorities into your schedule for the following day. This nightly ritual helps you start each day with a clear plan and a sense of purpose.

5. **Non-Negotiable Commitment.** Make your priorities non-negotiable. Understand that this may require time and prayer as you develop the discipline to consistently honor what's truly important. Your ultimate goal is to reach a place where you value yourself enough to prioritize what's essential for your well-being and purpose.

As you read on, you'll continue to learn how to prioritize your life so that you can do the things God has called you to do—after all, that's all you have time for. Everything else is just distractions that slow you down from fulfilling your assignment here on Earth. You'll also discover why being in good health must make your priority list.

Priority Quiz

This short quiz will help you understand God's order for prioritizing your life. It is a practical tool to help you assess your current priorities and understand how well they align with God's best for you.

How would you order the following?

- Time with God
- Your job/career/education
- Your family
- Your health/self-care
- Your ministry commitments

Soooooo, what did it look like? 1,3,2,5,4? 1,5,2,3,4?

And if you're really honest, it's 2,3,5,1,4. No matter how you slice it, many of us, and even more specifically, Christian women, continue to put themselves at the bottom of the list. We wear our busyness like a badge of honor. We're proud to brag about how busy we are. Meanwhile, deep down we're resentful, overstressed, overworked, and overweight. It's time to learn how to flip this badly flawed paradigm on its head and learn a Biblical framework for how you are to prioritize your life.

Ordering your Priorities

Now, it might already be obvious that God should be first in your life, but what about your second priority? What would you put after God? Your kids? Your ministry? Your husband? Here is where most of us begin to squirm. What if I told you that YOU should be second? I know what you're thinking…

Many of us were raised to think that putting ourselves before others is selfish and ungodly, but nothing could be further from the truth. Putting yourself first is one of the most selfless and Godly things you can do for yourself, your family, your boss, your church, and God.

First off, I want to be clear. The Bible does not lay out a hierarchical order for family relationship priorities. However, the scriptures give us some general principles for ordering our priorities.

Here's God's order for your priorities:

In your journey as a Christian, understanding and living by God's divine priorities can transform your life. Rather than viewing these priorities as rigid rules, consider them as a loving guide to help you lead a life full of purpose, love, and service.

1. Your Relationship with God: Your First and Most Precious Priority

   The foundation of it all begins with your relationship with God. As a Christian, making God your foremost priority is not a burden; it's an invitation to experience His unwavering love and guidance. When you center your life around Him, you align with His divine plan (Matthew 6:33; Mark 12:30; John 15:5). It's an opportunity to find your identity, your strength, and your peace in the embrace of your Heavenly Father.

2. Yourself: Embrace Your Worth as a Child of God

   Loving and caring for yourself is not selfish; it's an acknowledgment of your worth as a child of the Most High King. Recognize that by loving yourself, you equip yourself to love and serve others more fully. *You can be a bigger blessing if you're energized, happy, and healthy than if you're overworked, overweight, and resentful.*

   (Mark 12:31; Genesis 1:26; Psalms 139:14; 1 Corinthians 6:19).

3. Your Role as a Wife (if You're Married): Nurturing the "One Flesh" Bond

   For married women, the role of a wife holds a special place. Your relationship with your husband is an earthly reflection of God's love for the Church (Ephesians 5:22). It's about nurturing the "one flesh" bond, designed by God. The time you invest in your marriage strengthens this sacred connection and is an opportunity to experience God's love through your relationship.

4. Your Children: Cherishing God's Precious Gifts

Children, a beautiful result of the marital relationship, are precious gifts from the Lord (Psalms 127:3-5). They not only bring joy and love to your life but also serve as a reflection of spiritual truths about our relationship with our Heavenly Father (1 John 3:1). Your love for your children mirrors the love our Heavenly Father has for us. Cherish and nurture this bond with love and gratitude.

5. Your Work: Celebrate Your Contributions

    Work is a divine calling. In the book of Genesis, we see God planting a garden and putting Adam to work in it. When God viewed the fruits of His labor, He saw that it was "very good". Likewise, when you invest your efforts into your work, you are partaking in God's creative process. Take pride in your contributions, and know that when you do your work with excellence you mirror God's pleasure in His own creation.

6. Your Ministry: Embrace Your Calling to Serve

    We are all called to minister to others (1 Corinthians 12:7; 1 Peter 4:10-11). Serving others is a beautiful way to share God's love and grace. Your ministry, whether big or small, is an extension of His love in action. Embrace your calling to serve, and remember that your service is a testament to His boundless love.

7. Everything Else: Balance and Perspective

    Finally, as you navigate the various aspects of your life, remember that not everything can take the top spot. We've got to make tough choices. By aligning your priorities with God's loving order, you can create a balanced and fulfilling life. Everything else falls into place when you allow God's love and wisdom to guide your choices.

In embracing these priorities you'll discover a healthy life filled with love, purpose, and a deep connection to your Heavenly Father. Each step you take brings you closer to the plan He has for you. Embrace His priorities as an act of love for yourself, your loved ones, and your Heavenly Father.

Now, with this hierarchy in mind, ask yourself the following questions to see how you may need to adjust your priorities.

Your relationship with God

Is your life centered on God? The most effective and impactful thing we can do every day is to pursue continual communion with God. Although we may know that intellectually, many of us have a difficult time understanding just what that means. What does that look like in a practical sense?

Pursuing continual communion with God is not about following a rigid checklist of ten things, but rather a dynamic and personal journey. Here's what centering your life around God can look like in practical terms:

Continuous Conversation: Maintain an ongoing conversation with God throughout the day. Acknowledge His presence in your work, meals, walks, conversations, decision-making, parenting, and time with your spouse. Include Him in every aspect of your life.

Attitude of Gratitude: Cultivate a spirit of gratitude by giving thanks in everything. Recognize God's hand in both the ordinary and extraordinary moments of your life.

Scheduled Quiet Time: Set aside dedicated quiet time each day for deeper communion with God. This could include prayer, meditation, reading Scripture, or simply being still in His presence.

Obedience: Actively seek to do what God prompts you to do. Listen for His guidance and obey His leading in your life.

Prioritize His Will: Ask God to align your daily priorities with His will. Seek His guidance in decision-making and trust His direction.

Worship Throughout the Day: Look for opportunities to worship God as you go about your daily activities. Praise Him in your work, your relationships, and your daily experiences.

Self-Care: Honor your body as a temple of the Holy Spirit. Take care of yourself through proper rest, nutrition, and self-care practices.

Centering your life around God is a daily journey marked by a deepening relationship, trust, and obedience. It's about living in His presence, aligning your actions with His will, and sharing His love with the world around you.

Every other activity that you engage in should be done with this first priority in mind. As Colossians 3:17 teaches us, "And whatever you do, whether in word or deed, do it all in the name of the Lord Jesus, giving thanks to God the Father through him."

And just in case you're still unsure that God should be first and that everything we do should flow out of this priority, Mark 12:30 commands us to "Love the Lord your God with all your heart and with all your soul and with all your mind and with all your strength." All means just that! He wants us to give Him **all** we have. There's no room for half-hearted love or most-of-the-time love. Jesus reminds us that this is the most important commandment of all and it's not possible to be divided. "No one can serve two masters" (Matthew 6:24).

The final scripture I want us to look at is John 15:5: *"I am the vine; you are the branches. If you remain in me and I in you, you will bear much fruit; apart from me you can do nothing."*

Again, we see God's absolute truth. Apart from Him we can do NOTHING. We try our best to do it on our own, to do the right thing, to make wise decisions, to be self-controlled, and to be disciplined, but Jesus reminds us that apart from Him our efforts will always be unfruitful.

If God is not first in your life (and your health and weight loss efforts), you will not be successful.

When this relationship is in order, everything else will fall into place.

If this relationship is not where you want it to be, what can you do to begin to strengthen it?

Your relationship with yourself

Are you able to carve out time for self-care each day?

I understand that prioritizing oneself can be a challenging concept, particularly for many women, especially within the Christian faith, but this is crucial. It may initially appear self-serving, selfish, or even contrary to Christian values. However, it's essential to realize that this perspective is quite the opposite—it's deeply rooted in Christian principles.

Consider the safety instructions given on an airplane in the event of a loss of cabin pressure: "Put your own oxygen mask on first and then assist others."

143

Why this order? To put it plainly, you can't effectively help those in your care if you're not well yourself. The greatest act of care you can provide to those entrusted to your guidance is to ensure your own spiritual, physical, mental, and emotional health and well-being.

In nurturing and prioritizing yourself, you not only empower your ability to serve others but also exemplify a Christian virtue of self-care and self-love that aligns with God's desire for you to live a healthy and whole life.

If you don't look after your health, you will not be able to support your family, employees, students, parents, or anyone entrusted in your care to your full capacity. That's why you need to exercise and eat healthfully. If you don't nourish your mind, read books, keep learning and growing, you won't have the intellectual resources you need to share with others. If you don't get enough sleep, you won't have the patience, mental acuity, and strength to cope with life's daily challenges. If you don't take the time to get to the root of what keeps you stuck and emotionally bound, then you will never live the life of peace, freedom, and joy that Christ died for you to receive.

To confront this truth directly, it's important to acknowledge that consistently placing yourself at the bottom of your priority list can, in reality, be rooted in egotism and selfishness. Before passing judgment, consider the underlying motivations behind this behavior:

1. The belief that no one can do it as well as you can: This may stem from pride.

2. The need to make yourself indispensable: A manifestation of ego.

3. A desire for acknowledgment and recognition: Also tied to ego.

4. A belief that this is what it means to be a good wife, employee, or mother: Driven by fear.

5. A need to feel needed: Reflects fear and insecurity.

6. Being too afraid to say 'no' to others: A response to fear of judgment.

7. Identifying with the role of the 'go-to' person; fearing an identity crisis if you're not meeting everyone else's needs: Rooted in fear.

8. Not believing in what God wants of you: A spiritual disconnect.

9. Feeling unworthy: A self-worth issue.

10. Fearing rejection if you refuse others' requests: Fear-driven.

Recognizing these underlying motivations is crucial, and we'll spend quite a bit of time in Principle 12 talking more about fear. What I want you to grasp right now is that the urge to prioritize everything but ourselves can be misguided, turning what should be a blessing into a burden.

Reevaluating these motivations can lead to a more balanced and fulfilling life that aligns with God's intentions for you.

Get the picture? Too often our need to put other things before ourselves is grounded in the wrong motivation; therefore, instead of being a blessing, it's actually a curse.

To be clear, God does call us to be servants and givers, He calls us to be selfless. God calls us to care for the needy and to love our neighbor as ourselves. God calls us to deny ourselves and to care for our families. All very put-others-before-ourselves type of behaviors. So which is it? Do we put ourselves first or others first? On the surface it seems like a contradiction, but here's the caveat: Service, giving, and being a blessing are selfless acts, but only when they come from a place of love, not legalism, pleasing others or checking these duties off a list. If we truly understand God's message, His assumption is that we already love ourselves.

Unfortunately, this is not the case for many women. We don't love ourselves, we don't feel worthy of love, and we don't see ourselves in God's image. That's why we confuse self-care with being selfish.

If we don't give from a place of love then it's our egos that are running the show and it shows up as fear, insecurity, pressure, people-pleasing, and martyrdom.

Let's turn to the Word of God to gain insight into the framework and context of loving others. In Mark 12:31, we find a teachable moment where religious leaders sought to test Jesus by asking Him to identify the greatest commandment among all the laws. His response was beautifully simple: Love God and love others.

According to Jesus, these two commandments capture the essence of the entire Decalogue. However, a crucial aspect often goes unnoticed: "Love your neighbor as yourself." This implied that we already love ourselves, and not in the superficial "I just treated myself to ice cream" manner but in a deeper way, akin to the love God demonstrates toward us.

So, on a scale of 1 to 10, how much do you genuinely love yourself? If your self-love score isn't as favorable as it should be, then how can you authentically love others, a commandment deemed as one of the greatest? It all starts with you. Do you believe that you can do all things through Christ? Do you believe in your true identity as created in God's image, as Genesis 1:26 teaches?

To be created in God's image means having dominion over everything, including our minds (Philippians 4:8), bodies (1 Corinthians 9:27), and emotions (Philippians 4:6). We are called to walk in righteousness and holiness (Ephesians 4:24).

Psalms 139:14 beautifully proclaims, "I praise you because I am fearfully and wonderfully made; your works are wonderful, I know that full well" (NIV). This verse reminds us that God meticulously crafted each of us with tender, loving care. Consider the care you bestow upon the things you hold most precious in your life. That's how you should begin to think of yourself and treat yourself. You are indeed God's masterpiece (Ephesians 2:10).

The more you recognize yourself as God's masterpiece, the more you'll acknowledge that your ability to love others is intrinsically tied to how you love yourself. This realization should inspire you to diligently practice self-care. Self-care replenishes your spiritual, mental, and emotional reserves, creating the space in your life to fulfill the Biblical commandment of loving others as you love yourself.

Your role as wife and mother

As women, we have the blessing (which can sometimes feel like a curse) of meeting the emotional needs of our entire family. We are blessed with the ability to remember our mother-in-law's birthday and always find the perfect gift for her; shop for all of the Christmas gifts every year; organize all the birthday parties; shop for everyone's clothes—including your husband's; organize all of the medical appointments, school trips, and budget; stay up to date on what's happening in the lives of all of your children's friends; make sure everyone is on time and looking half-decent for church each Sunday, etc.

This incredible responsibility often takes on two extremes: 1. We devote all of our time, effort, and attention to our family to the exclusion of ourselves. We put so much energy into our children that we leave nothing for ourselves. 2. Being a good wife and mother becomes our main identity, so we don't develop ourselves much beyond that.

We're so tired from working outside the home or we're so worn out from doing so much for them that we become resentful, bitter, and downright mean.

God wants us to have a healthy balanced approach when it comes to our families.

The Book of Proverbs provides a beautiful example of what it means to be a Godly wife and mother. Although we get a picture of a hard-working woman, it also tells us that, "She dresses herself with strength and makes her arms strong" (Proverbs 31:17). This implies that she practices self-care. She is not haggard and worn out, and seems to delight in what she does for her family. Can you say the same? Do you delight in taking care of your family's needs? Or are you so tired that it's easier to just order pizza for everyone and veg out in front of Netflix?

Are you available for them, or are you busy working or doing things for others? Is your home in order? Can they look to you as a model of health? Do you have any gas left in your tank at the end of the day for your children, and especially your husband? As women of God, we want to model how to take care of ourselves so that the people under our influence will take care of themselves.

Your relationship with work/ministry

Are you working wholeheartedly as unto the Lord as Scripture instructs us? (Ephesians 6:7; 1 Corinthians 12:7; 1 Peter 4:10-11)

In the realm of work, whether you operate from a physical workplace or not, whether you're a student or enjoying retirement, it's easy to become ensnared by the relentless pursuit of long, stress-filled hours each day, turning our work into an idol.

In the New Testament church, leaders were required to demonstrate faithfulness at home *before* they were considered eligible for leadership (Titus 1:5-9, 1 Timothy 3:1-13).

Management of your household comes before caring for God's church. Your household comes first because it is the proving ground for your ministry. Your household also comes first because anyone who does not provide for his household is worse than an unbeliever (1 Timothy 5:8).

Many well-intended people believe that their work or ministry should come before themselves or their family, but that is simply not the case. God has called us to work/to serve and to minister to others. Sometimes it will require you to sacrifice in other areas of your life, but this should be temporary. If a lot of time is spent with work/ministry, is your family or husband on board? Have you talked to them about it? Are you able to still take care of yourself and your family? If your work is keeping you from your higher priorities, then it's time to reassess.

If we allow the Holy Spirit to order our steps and strip everything else away so that we're left with a schedule based on God's priorities, wisdom and leading, we will be able to experience the divine health He created for us to enjoy.

Managing Your Schedule

> *"But first and most importantly seek (aim at, strive after) His kingdom and His righteousness [His way of doing and being right—the attitude and character of God], and all these things will be given to you also."* (Matthew 6:33 AMP)

In his Sermon on the Mount in the Gospel of Matthew, Jesus addressed a multitude of enlightening topics that resonated with the crowds. He touched upon matters like lust, divorce, vows, revenge, love for one's enemies, giving to the needy, prayer, fasting, and the role of money. These teachings provide valuable insights into life's priorities, and it's particularly crucial to understand them in the context of our health.

Worry, a prevalent issue in our lives, often leads us astray, causing us to chase daily emergencies rather than focusing on God's intended priorities. Worry fosters self-sufficiency, making us believe we can handle everything without relying on God.

However, Jesus imparts a simple yet profound truth amidst these teachings: "Seek the Kingdom of God above all else, and live righteously, and he will give you everything you need" (Matthew 6:33, NLT). This powerful statement reminds us that seeking God's kingdom and aligning with His righteousness should be at the forefront of our priorities, including our health.

This truth isn't a formula for amassing riches or achieving the perfect body. Instead, it's a description of how God operates in our lives. By understanding His ways, we can stop wasting time and energy on trivial worries and instead embrace the life God has called us to lead.

Prioritizing our health is an integral part of seeking God's kingdom first. Just as we're not called to do everything in life, God hasn't called us to neglect our health. He desires that we excel in a few important areas, and one of these areas should unquestionably be our well-being.

The challenge we face is often not whether to invest in our health over other pursuits, but rather how to integrate healthy habits into our daily lives amidst our busy schedules.

Questions like:

- "Where do I fit exercise into a day where I already wake up at 5:00 am to prepare lunches and get everyone organized?"

- "How can I even think of grocery shopping when I've got 20 people waiting for me at work?"

- "How do I make the time to prepare nutritious foods when the entire Sunday School department is relying on me to show up?"

I don't doubt that you sincerely want to be healthier, but when the pressure of fitting 10 seemingly urgent things into your day confronts you, it's your health that most often gets squeezed out. You don't want to neglect your health, but you just feel like you don't have any other choice.

Your daily priorities may always take precedence over your health. Other priorities will also be imposed, such as work/school needs, taking the kids to their games, or shopping for a friend's birthday, wedding, or housewarming gift—priorities you impose on yourself or are imposed on you. And unless exercise and taking the time to eat healthily are high on your priority list, odds are they will constantly fall off your daily to-do list.

Perhaps you're not even aware of what your priorities are, so getting clarity and giving them a hierarchy of most to least important as you did in the last chapter will greatly help to move you from a place of stress and frustration to calm planning.

Good health can have a positive trickle-down effect on your other priorities. After all, what area of your life wouldn't benefit from you having more energy, feeling super-charged, and positive about yourself? When you take the time to really understand what your priorities are and put them into a logical order, health always gets moved up in priority. It just makes sense.

Even still, there will be days where your health goals are getting pushed out by other priorities. But what if you did not have to choose between your health and your other priorities? What if you could have them both?

You can always find creative ways to fit your health goals in. For example, at work you can choose to take the stairs (or some of them) instead of the elevator, or do some light exercises right at your desk or go for a walk while on break. If you're with your kids, you can engage them in physical activities that you can all do together or prepare fun, healthful meals for everyone. Similar ideas if you're volunteering at church or for other causes, or doing your chores.

When you understand where your health and weight-releasing goals fit into your schedule, your mind begins to constantly look for ways to fulfill that need and you'll begin to naturally and automatically make healthier choices from a place of self-love and not a place of 'should-do' or 'need to'.

In his book *The Purpose Driven Life*, Pastor Rick Warren emphasizes an impactful insight: "You have just enough time to do God's will. If you can't get it all done, it means you're trying to do more than God intended for you to do." Does this resonate with your life story? Are you possibly attempting to shoulder too many responsibilities or investing your time in the wrong pursuits? While many of us grasp the importance of prioritizing our lives, the essential question remains: Do you truly trust God enough to believe that He will guide your steps and arrange your schedule according to His divine plan? If your desire is to embrace a healthier lifestyle but you find it challenging to make time for it, consider pondering the following questions, keeping God's perspective in mind.

Time Management Quiz

1. Is the amount of time you spend on other priorities in line with their level of priority? (e.g. Are you spending too much time on low priorities, instead of addressing high priorities?)

2. Look at priorities that take up a lot of your time. Are you confident that God has called you to spend your time on them?

3. Have you prayed about your workload and asked God to help you order your steps?

4. Do you feel like you are led by the Spirit and therefore work with ease, or do you constantly feel under pressure to get things done? Are you always behind?

5. Do you spend time in your morning in prayer before you start managing the other priorities of the day?

6. Are you able to carve out at least one hour in the day for self-care, which includes looking after your health?

7. Have you been hearing messages, signs, hints, or warnings about your health, yet you neglect to take action?

8. If someone asks you to do something that will require a lot of your time, do you pray about it first?

9. Are you able to focus on your priorities instead of dealing with urgent matters (putting out fires)?

10. Do you understand the impact that being healthy will have on your ministry, calling, or other priorities?

As you reflect on these important questions in the time management quiz, remember that aligning your priorities with God's will and perspective will make all the difference. If you found yourself answering 'no' to any of these questions, it's an opportunity to take a deeper look at your priorities, your schedule, and your health, and align them with God's divine plan.

There should be no question in your mind that God wants you to be healthy. His Word has made that clear many times over (3 John 1:2, 1 Cor. 6:19-20, John 10:10). How will you align your priorities with God's?

As you move forward, consider this: If you allow the Holy Spirit to strip everything else away so that you're left with a schedule based on God's priorities, wisdom and guidance, you will ultimately experience the divine health that He intended for you to enjoy. So, embrace this journey with faith and commitment, for in doing so you'll find fulfillment, purpose, and a healthier, more abundant life in His divine presence and purpose.

Principle 10 Summary

Reflect on these key points:

- Prioritize God as the highest and most important aspect of your life, aligning your daily actions and choices with His will.

- Place yourself as the second priority, understanding that self-care is essential for serving others effectively and fulfilling your God-given roles.

- Ensure your daily schedule reflects these priorities, seeking ways to integrate health and self-care into your life, ultimately aligning with God's plan for your well-being.

Principle #11: Align Your Health with Your Values

Live in Alignment

In our *Weight Loss, God's Way* program, when we ask women if they feel they live their life in integrity, most of them say 'yes'. But when asked about their integrity concerning their health choices there's often some uncertainty, hesitation, or even unease. It's an intriguing observation, isn't it? Why is it that integrity, a virtue often linked with honesty and steadfastness in one's values and deeds, appears to slip away when it comes to making choices about our health?

In this chapter, we'll explore how Principle #11—Integrity and Values—can be another guiding light in your journey. Integrity, I define as believing, thinking, and acting in alignment with who God created you to be. This encompasses your God-given personality, interests, values, and strengths.

Living in integrity means that you conduct yourself in a manner consistent with your innermost values and beliefs. When you do, everything feels right and you experience inner peace, productivity, motivation, and inspiration to be the best version of yourself.

Imagine a life where your health choices seamlessly align with your values. In such a scenario, being healthy isn't a chore or a constant battle but rather a natural extension of who you are as a woman of God.

The word "integrity" itself is derived from the same Latin root as "integer", which means whole or not divided. In the realm of mathematics integers are whole numbers, not fractions. It's a powerful analogy for our lives. God created us as whole beings—body, soul, and spirit. Living with integrity means that all aspects of ourselves operate in unison and harmony. This alignment is beautifully expressed in 3 John 2 (KJV): "*Beloved, I wish above all things that thou mayest prosper and be in health, even as thy soul prospereth,*" highlighting that health encompass the physical, spiritual, and emotional aspects of our lives.

The Book of Proverbs is a treasure trove of wisdom on living lives of value and integrity. Consider these verses:

> - *Proverbs 10:9 (NIV): "Whoever walks in integrity walks securely, but whoever takes crooked paths will be found out."*
>
> - *Proverbs 11:3 (NIV): "The integrity of the upright guides them, but the unfaithful are destroyed by their duplicity."*
>
> - *Proverbs 20:7 (NKJV): "The righteous man walks in his integrity; His children are blessed after him."*
>
> - *Proverbs 19:1 (ESV): "Better is a poor person who walks in his integrity than one who is crooked in speech and is a fool."*

These proverbs, penned by King Solomon, provide practical advice for living a life of value and integrity. King Solomon, renowned as one of the wisest men to have ever lived, intended these proverbs to help readers apply the fear of the Lord to their lives, seeing situations through God's perspective.

Living with integrity, especially regarding your health, involves incorporating your God-given personality, interests, values, and strengths into your daily choices. When these factors aren't considered, everything feels like a struggle and an effort. You may find it challenging to motivate yourself to stay committed to health goals because the way you're approaching them may be out of alignment with your values.

Picture a life where the pursuit of health and well-being isn't a constant struggle but a natural, harmonious extension of your identity as a devoted woman or man of God. It is possible. To help you get there, you're going to first have to understand and align with your core values.

Begin by taking a reflective journey into your own heart. Ask yourself what truly matters to you and why. What are the driving forces behind your daily choices and actions? These are your values, the deep-seated principles that form the core of your character and influence your every decision. It's time to explore if these values are in perfect harmony with your life's purpose and goals. Later in this chapter, you'll review an extensive list of values to help you get clear on what your values are, but for now let me continue to paint the picture.

Imagine your values as the ingredients in a recipe. When your values complement your health goals, you create a delicious and harmonious dish. If your values clash with your objectives it's like mixing incompatible flavors, resulting in a less-than-appetizing meal. Yet, this is what we often do when we commit to getting healthier. We throw in a little of what we saw on You-Tube, with a bit of information that our friend told us with a bit of what we watched on the hit show *The Biggest Loser* back in the day, and the next thing you know we've got a hodge-podge of conflicting ingredients in our recipe for health. It's as if we're trying to make a gourmet meal with items that simply don't go together. This mishmash of advice and strategies can leave us feeling overwhelmed and disheartened, like trying to savor a dish with clashing flavors. Instead, to create a recipe for success in your health journey, it's essential to carefully select and combine the right ingredients that align with your unique values. This way, you can craft a health plan that's not only effective but also personally fulfilling, just like a well-prepared, delectable meal that leaves you satisfied and content.

Your values are unique to you, and living in alignment with them is what brings about lasting changes. This newfound clarity will simplify your life. Aligning your health with your values will help you gain an understanding of what truly matters so you can discard the noise that previously cluttered your decision-making. No longer are you weighed down by inner conflicts and doubts. Instead, you find yourself walking a path illuminated by a guiding light that's in alignment with God's truth.

The Word of God also tells us that:

Integrity is valued more than wealth (Proverbs 22:1, 16:8).

In a world full of gray areas, it can be difficult to walk in integrity. In fact, people who often walk the 'straight and narrow' are often ridiculed in society. As usual, God's Word causes us to reprioritize what we deem important. Integrity should be one of the virtues we seek after.

Integrity has generational blessings (long-lasting implications). "The righteous man walks in his integrity; His children are blessed after him" Proverbs 20:7 (NKJV). Children learn from what they see. We learned how to behave from watching our parents. When we walk in integrity we pass that blessing on to our children, and they pass it on to their children.

It provides guidance and direction. Proverbs 11:3 (NIV): "The integrity of the upright guides them, but the unfaithful are destroyed by their duplicity." When you lack integrity, you will do whatever it takes to have what you want, even when it's wrong. Solomon teaches us that if you are following after the Lord, walking in integrity, you will go where He leads you, and it will lead to blessings.

It simplifies life. There is no substitute for the freedom, peace, and joy that comes from living from your values. Having a lens through which you can filter everything simplifies life. Instead of always worrying about whether you're doing the right thing, over-concerned about people-pleasing or trying to live up to some false expectations, living from your values helps keep your mind at peace.

Integrity in Honoring Your Body

Earlier, we defined integrity as believing, thinking, and acting in alignment with who God created you to be. Or, put another way, we can use Philippians 4:8 to define it as a life consumed with thinking (and, acting) on "whatever is true, whatever is noble, whatever is right, whatever is pure, whatever is lovely, whatever is admirable" (NIV).

With this definition in mind, ask yourself, do you live in integrity each day? When we live our daily lives in alignment with our values, things feel right; we feel at peace and we are productive, motivated, and inspired to be our best.

It's been said that you may be the only bible that some people ever read.

Meaning, when people look at your life, do they see Christ in you? Do your actions lead them to want to become a Christian?

This can feel like a very heavy weight and burden, and if you're not mindful you can let the enemy have a field day with this thought. Conversely, you would be naive if you pretended that people are not looking at what you do and judging your faith. They want to know if Christianity is real or fake, and your actions or inactions can either draw them closer to the gospel or repel them. Whether you like it or not, people will make value judgments based on your actions. This requires an honest examination of your life. Are you living in integrity with the gospel in all areas of your life?

The point here is to not to strive for perfection, nor is it to try to please anyone. In fact, it's the exact opposite. Your only desire should be to please Christ (Gal 1:10) and it is when you please Him that you are representing your faith well.

When many of us look at our lives, we think we're pretty honest. For the most part, we probably don't steal (at least anything significant), we definitely don't murder anyone (if bugs don't count), and we don't covet our neighbor's spouse (other things…well maybe).

In his book *Who You Are When No One's Looking: Choosing Consistency, Resisting Compromise*, Bill Hybels offers an interesting insight into human behavior and character. He emphasizes that most of us tend to be on our best behavior when we're aware of being watched, such as in social settings or when others are present. We put on a facade, projecting our ideal self, making sure we act in ways that align with societal expectations and norms.

However, the true measure of one's character lies in those moments when no one is looking, when there are no external eyes to impress. It's in the quiet, private moments when our integrity is tested. Do we uphold the same standards and values when there's no audience? This is where the essence of integrity comes into play.

Let me share a couple of chuckle-worthy glimpses into a real life experiences from several years ago. Picture this: I'm at a restaurant with friends or family, and I decide to order the virtuous, garden-fresh salad. Why? Well, it's all about putting on a show, creating the illusion of a health-conscious guru in front of my companions. I want them to think, "Wow, look at Cathy, making those stellar food choices!" But, here's the twist. The moment I stepped foot inside my home, it was like a switch flipped and I made a beeline for the leftover pizza or whatever tantalizing snacks were stashed away in the pantry. It's as if the absence of an audience gave me a golden ticket to indulge in less-than-saintly culinary delights.

And, hold on to your hats for this one. I recall that time I had just returned from McDonald's with my son. As I spotted someone I knew, I didn't just say hello; oh no, I decided to pull off a covert operation. I dove into the bushes, hiding like a burger bandit on the run for fear that they would see my McDonald's bag.

But you see, the real comedy lies in the question: am I committed to a healthy lifestyle, even when no one's peeking over my shoulder? Or am I drawn into the irresistible charm of less-than-angelic eating habits once the curtains close? Laughter aside, it's a test of integrity and a reminder that being the same person in public and in private takes a blend of commitment, honesty, and a dash of humor.

Integrity, in the context of my health journey, means being unwavering in my choices regardless of whether anyone is watching. It's about aligning my actions with my values and convictions, even when I'm the only one holding myself accountable. And to do this effectively, I've come to understand that I need God's guidance and strength as my constant companion. It's through His presence in my life that I've learned to make consistent, health-conscious decisions both in public and in private, honoring my commitment to a healthy and God-honoring lifestyle.

This doesn't mean that I never indulge in the occasional treat or enjoy a less nutritious meal. It's about understanding that even when I do, it's done from a place of integrity. In other words, I'm not deceiving myself or going against my own values. It's a conscious choice I make, and I'm fully aware of the decision, taking responsibility for it. This level of honesty and self-awareness is an essential part of living with integrity, especially when it comes to my health choices.

This virtue is not something that can be mastered by sheer willpower or self-discipline alone. It requires the guidance and strength that come from consistently surrendering everything and everyone to God. When you're aware of God's presence in your life and make choices with the knowledge that He is always watching, it becomes a powerful motivator for maintaining integrity.

Developing and living with integrity is a continuous journey. It involves self-reflection, accountability to a higher standard, a commitment to living in a way that honors your core values and beliefs, and a whole lot of grace. With God's guidance and strength you can strive to be the same person in public and in private, consistently upholding the principles and values that reflect who you are as a child of God.

So, in the context of your health journey, integrity means not only making healthy choices when others are watching but also when you are alone. It means that your commitment to a healthy lifestyle isn't just for show, but a genuine expression of your values and respect for the body God has entrusted

> **So, in the context of your health journey, integrity means not only making healthy choices when others are watching but also when you are alone.**

to you. By living with integrity, you honor God's creation and your commitment to being the best version of yourself, whether in public or in private.

Barb Raveling's book *Taste for Truth* delves deep into the psychological and spiritual aspects of the battle for better health. One of the key insights she presents is the concept that the strongholds, those recurring patterns of unhealthy behaviors, are often rooted in lies. While on the surface this idea might seem overly simplistic, it carries meaningful significance in the context of our health and wellness journey.

Consider the common lies that we tell ourselves when it comes to our health. These falsehoods often lurk beneath the surface, subtly influencing our choices and behaviors. We might say, "One bite won't hurt," convincing ourselves that a small indulgence won't have significant consequences. However, deep down, we know that "one bite is too much, and a thousand is never enough."

Another lie we frequently encounter is the belief that a certain food will make us feel better. Emotional eating often hinges on this idea that certain comfort foods can provide solace or relief from life's stress and emotional challenges. Yet, in reality, we often end up feeling worse after indulging in these temporary comforts.

Then there's the common excuse, "I've given it to the Lord," which sometimes masks a lack of genuine spiritual connection. Surrendering your health to God entails more than just superficial prayers or fleeting commitments. It involves wholehearted submission of your desires, challenges, and goals to His divine guidance.

The classic "I'll start on Monday" lie is a perpetual temptation for many. We often convince ourselves that we'll make healthier choices tomorrow or in the future, but the truth is, "It's Now O'clock." Waiting for a specific day to start making a difference in your health journey only postpones the progress you can achieve today.

"I had no choice" is another deceptive statement we use to justify unhealthy decisions. We might convince ourselves that there were no better options, but in reality we could have made a healthier choice if we had truly wanted to. This is often reflected in moments when we claim there's nothing else to eat, when in fact we simply didn't want to choose the available healthier options.

And then there's the perpetual procrastination with "I'll exercise later." This lie often leads to inaction and the deferral of our health goals to an unspecified future date.

Lastly, some might downplay the importance of their health with the declaration, "I don't care what I look like." However, this can be a form of self-deception, as our health significantly impacts our overall well-being, both physically and emotionally.

Barb Raveling's insight highlights the complexity of the battle for better health. These lies, though seemingly simple, have a major impact on our choices and habits. Recognizing and challenging these lies will help you break free from strongholds and achieve a healthier and more fulfilling life. In the coming chapters, you'll learn how to replace these lies with the truth of your values and convictions and ultimately living a life of integrity and honesty, even in your health.

Becoming a person of integrity means understanding that every choice you make, even in the privacy of your own thoughts, carries real consequences for your overall well-being. I'm not talking solely about changing your habits; it's about ensuring that your actions align with your deeply held values and beliefs. In doing so, you can liberate yourself from the strongholds that may have hindered your progress, embracing a life marked by consistency and honesty, even when you believe no one is watching.

Next you'll explore, clarify, and prioritize your values so that your life is in harmony with them. This process will empower you to live with integrity and authenticity, aligning your choices with your deepest desires.

Living in Alignment with your Values

To recap, living in integrity is about embracing your unique God-given personality, interests, values, and strengths. The more you align your life with these aspects, the more you'll experience joy, peace, and freedom. It's common to simply go through the motions day by day without ever considering these factors. You might sense that something feels "off", but the reasons remain elusive. You might have made a commitment to get healthier by downloading meal plans and workout routines from the internet, only to find yourself bored, frustrated, or overwhelmed shortly after beginning. This could be a sign that your approach is not in harmony with your values.

When you can successfully live in accordance with your values, being healthy ceases to be a burden or a chore. Instead, it naturally becomes an extension of who you are as a woman of God. But before reaching that point, you'll need to know what your values are.

For example, if you're a creative person, explore activities that nurture your creativity in the context of health. You might experiment with creating nutritious and visually appealing meals, turning your kitchen into a canvas for culinary art. If you value enjoyment, seek ways to make your health journey joyful. This could involve incorporating enjoyable exercises like dancing to your favorite music, ensuring that your path to better health is filled with moments of happiness. Consider the gratitude you feel after a rejuvenating workout, the peace that accompanies a mindful walk in nature, or the faith that empowers you to stay committed to your health goals. These are moments of alignment with your values in the context of your health journey.

Hint: Living by your values will leave little room for worrying or obsessing about your weight. Therefore, let's pray for the desire to do more of what we love every day!

Complete Your Values Assessment

There are many different values assessments on the market. This one I've put together myself over the year taking a little bit from here and a little bit from there. To complete the assessment, take a moment to review the list of values and select the ones that resonate with you. As you examine your life and consider the values that are most important to you, think about whether your daily actions align with these values either in your health or in your life in general. Your struggles and discomfort often signal that you're not living in alignment with your core values, which can lead to feelings of discontent, despair, discouragement, disappointment, and even depression.

To determine your values effectively, start by scanning a list of values to get a sense of the wide range of options. Select 10 values that resonate with you the most. Once you've identified these 10 values, take the next step of narrowing them down to your top five, the values that truly define and guide your life. As a bonus exercise, you might even seek out scripture that emphasizes these values.

Abundance	Fun	Recognition
Achievement	Goodwill	Prosperity
Adventure	Gratitude	Punctuality
Ambition	Harmony	Reliability
Beauty	Honesty	Respect
Calm	Honor	Reputation
Challenge	Humility	Responsiveness
Charity	Independence	Safety
Cleanliness	Individuality	Security
Community	Integrity	Serenity
Communication	Intensity	Service
Connection	Joy	Simplicity

Cooperation	Justice	Sophistication
Creativity	Kindness	Speed
Daring	Knowledge	Spirituality
Decisiveness	Leadership	Stability
Democracy	Love	Status
Discovery	Loyalty	Strength
Diversity	Magnificence	Success
Efficiency	Meaning	Teamwork
Equality	Money	Timeliness
Excellence	Openness	Tolerance
Enjoyment	Order	Tradition
Faith	Patriotism	Tranquility
Excitement	Peace	Truth
Fairness	Pleasure	Variety
Family Unity	Power	Wealth
Flair	Practicality	Wisdom
Freedom	Privacy	
Friendship	Progress	

If you're finding it challenging to narrow down your values, consider using the following questions to help you:

1. Peak Experiences

   Think of a past experience when you were fully engaged with your values. How did it feel? What specific values were you honoring during that time?

2. Suppressed Values

   Recall a time when you were not living in alignment with your values and, as a result, you felt discouraged, disappointed, frustrated, or angry. What value was being suppressed or ignored during that period?

3. Daily Behaviors

Reflect on your daily behaviors or habits that support your values. What are the actions you consistently take to honor your core values?

4. Non-Supportive Behaviors

Identify three non-supportive behaviors or habits that you regularly engage in, which are outside your core values. These behaviors can also provide insight into what you truly value and what might be misaligned in your life.

This process will bring a new level of clarity to your decision-making process in the context of your health and weight release journey. Pay attention to how aligned your daily actions are with your values. This awareness can be particularly beneficial if consistency and honesty are high on your list of values. With the guidance of the Holy Spirit, your values will encourage you to choose activities that resonate with your character. For example, you might find yourself inclined to exercise by walking with a friend rather than joining a gym because you highly value friendship and communication. Your values bring a sense of clarity and simplicity to your health journey, helping you identify the activities, behaviors, and decisions that align with who you truly are.

As we conclude this chapter, remember that living with integrity on your health journey is a journey of self-awareness, honesty, and alignment with your core values. It's a commitment to make choices that honor not only your physical well-being but also your beliefs and deepest desires. By choosing to be the same person in public and in private, consistently upholding your values and principles, you create a testimony to your faith and integrity. Your journey is a reflection of who you are as a child of God, making every step a testament to your commitment to live in authenticity and honesty.

Principle 11 Summary

Reflect on these key points:

- Integrity challenges us to be the same person at home as we are in public. How do you live when no one is watching?

- Whether you're the leader of a country or a stay-at-home mom, God expects the same level of integrity from all of us.

- When you live in integrity with your values, you are not led by what you're feeling but by God's universal truths and principles such as the laws of reaping and sowing.

- Integrity does not believe in the gray area but believes in following God's truths and principles rather than the crowd.

Principle #12: Get to the Root of Why You Do What You Do

Develop The Courage to Change

Can you relate to this scenario?

You wake up feeling good. "It's going to be a great day," you tell yourself. You only hit the snooze button once, pray, and head to the bathroom for your morning routine. You make conscious choices for your health, exercise, and prepare nourishing meals. You move through your day with intention, prioritizing your health at every turn. And then, seemingly out of nowhere, it happens: you sabotage yourself. You pass by the bowl of treats always sitting at the front desk at your workplace and grab a handful; you end up eating all the kids' leftovers; you end up going out to eat after church and throw caution to the wind. It's as if a switch flips, and you find yourself making choices that directly contradict your earlier intentions. You're left bewildered, questioning why you would undermine the very goals you hold dear.

This experience, as confounding as it is, is very common. It's a narrative that many of us can relate to, and it echoes the sentiments of the apostle Paul in Romans 7:15. He, too, grappled and lamented with an inner conflict, a struggle between his conscious desires and his inexplicable actions. His words, "For what I am doing, I do not understand. For what I will to do, that I do not practice; but what I hate, that I do" (NKJV), resonate with a deep sense of confusion and frustration.

My heartfelt hope is that you will apprehend this dream-robber that dwells in the hidden recesses of your mind. It is elusive yet profoundly influential.

It quietly and seductively steers your actions and informs your choices. At the very core of many of these self-sabotaging behaviors stands a formidable and omnipresent force: fear.

Understanding the role of fear in your journey is a crucial step towards breaking free from its grasp. Your next step in this journey will be to shine light on those dark corners of your psyche where fear resides, bringing them into the open, bringing them under subjection to God. This process can be both enlightening and liberating as you confront fear head-on and make conscious choices for your health that align with what you most desire.

To truly comprehend the insidiousness of fear, let us journey back to the idyllic Garden of Eden. Prior to the fall, Adam walked freely in perfect fellowship with God. But after the fall, sin entered the world and, with it, it's companion fear. Fear is the result of separation from the love of God (1 John 4:18). Notice that Adam and Eve only felt fear after Satan planted a seed in their minds that they might be lacking something. And after sinning, it was fear that had them hide from God when He called them.

> *"He answered, "I heard you in the garden, and I was afraid because I was naked; so I hid.""" (Genesis 3:10 NIV)*

This same fear that took hold of our ancestors continues to sabotage us today. Its subtle goal is to keep us from experiencing deep fellowship and union with God that we were created for. If we are not proactive in addressing it, the voice of fear can become so deafening that we risk becoming desensitized to the gentle whisper of God's guidance.

In times when fear appears to hold us captive, let these words be a source of encouragement: even when it doesn't always feel like it, the Bible reassures us that nothing can ultimately separate us from the boundless love of God (Romans 8:35-37).

In his book *Faith and Food*, Norman Wirzba, an esteemed professor of Christian Theology at Duke Divinity School, puts forth a thought-provoking perspective:

"The root of all sin is fear: the profound apprehension that we are insignificant; the inner drive, consequently, to craft an ego-boosting facsimile of ourselves to venerate, to put our faith in these self-constructed illusions—our fabricated selves. I believe that all sins ultimately stem from a lack of realism; even the ordinary, day-to-day transgressions of the flesh, seemingly born from mere childish desires, ultimately trace back to a deep-seated anxiety about our own worth, an anxiety that drives us to seek self-reassurance."

Professor Wirzba's statement echoes the wisdom found in Psalms 139:23-24, where David earnestly implores God to search into the depths of his innermost thoughts, seeking to reveal any offensive aspects. Within these coming pages, you are encouraged to make a similar plea to the Almighty. Here, you will humbly request that He search your heart as you relinquish control of the steering wheel in your journey that steers your health and weight loss efforts. You will extend an invitation to the Lord to take the helm, allowing Him to enter your life and combat the fears that threaten to smother your personal growth at its very core.

As you allow God to perform this exploratory surgery of your heart like David did, He will unveil the true cravings that perpetuate your anxieties and hinder your progress, gently guiding you back towards His perfect love, which has the power to dispel all fear (1 John 4:18). Remember, God is your Creator, and His understanding of you far exceeds your own. Therefore, it is not only logical but also wise to seek His guidance rather than relying solely on your own limited understanding.

The remainder of this book will explore how these fears have taken root in your life and how they have sought to constrict and smother your growth, obstructing you from yielding a bountiful harvest. You will learn how to exercise authority over your fears, drawing inspiration from Genesis 1:28, where the Divine directive is to have dominion. By doing so your fears will become allies in your journey toward health, rather than continuing to serve as saboteurs.

So as you journey through the pages ahead, be prepared to unearth the depths of your fears, acknowledge their influence, and transform them into powerful allies on your path to better health and wellness.

It still may be hard for you to grasp right now, so it's worth repeating, fear (when unsurrendered) is at the root of why you've been spinning your wheels.

It's the root cause of why you wake up in the morning and decide to eat healthy but end up having McDonald's for dinner.

It's the root cause of why you put on your gym clothes to work out but end up on the couch, binge-watching TV.

And it's the root cause of why you have a disagreement with your spouse and end up eating the entire container of ice cream.

Fear Defined

You may be familiar with this acronyms for fear.

F.E.A.R.

False

Evidence

Appearing

Real

Fear can be both real and perceived. It's prudent to pay attention to real fears such as walking too close to the edge of a cliff or staying clear of a bees' nest. But you also possess many perceived fears you need to be aware of. They are not dangerous in and of themselves but they appear real and can sabotage, paralyze, and do some real damage in life if you're not vigilant. Some fears strike right to the core of your being. They are universal and hard-wired into us for survival. They are known as core fears.

Core fears are your deepest negative emotional response to perceived threat or danger. They include fear of failure, extinction (injury or death), loss of autonomy or control, separation, abandonment, rejection, humiliation, shame, and worthlessness.

I've read that the term 'Fear not' is the most repeated command in the Bible (Exodus 20:20, Joshua 1:9, Isaiah 41:10, Psalms 34:4, Phil 4:4-7 to name just a few), so your ability to keep them from sabotaging you must be important to God. After all, He would never command you to do something that He has not enabled you to do (Isaiah 41:19). So let's get busy learning how to release your fears to God. Scripture tells us that you are called to have dominion over everything. This includes fear. It is an emotion programmed into the nervous system, which, like all emotions, are created to serve us, not the other way around since you are called to have dominion over everything (Psalms 8:6).

Fears are instinctual and serve as protective mechanisms. They show up in our lives to guard us from danger and harm. Fear demands a response or reaction; for example, it prompts us to run or freeze when we sense impending danger. Interestingly, in the animal kingdom, some creatures like the opossum fake their own death when they sense fear as a strategy to escape predators. When an opossum encounters a predator or perceives imminent danger it goes into a state of tonic immobility, which closely resembles death. During this state, it becomes limp and unresponsive, with its body going limp, its mouth hanging open, and its tongue lolling out. It may even emit a foul-smelling fluid from its anal glands, further contributing to the illusion of being a rotting carcass. While we might not go to quite the same lengths as our furry friend, understanding our own fear responses can certainly help us navigate life's challenges with a bit more grace and understanding.

Beyond physical safety, fear fosters caution and prevents us from taking unnecessary risks, whether crossing a busy street or handling hazardous materials. It maintains social harmony by making us mindful of social consequences like embarrassment or rejection. Fear can also serves as a moral compass, guiding us away from unethical choices. Additionally, fear discourages recklessness and promotes thoughtful decision-making, while fostering emotional and financial well-being. So if fear is such a good thing, why has it gotten such a bad rap as I laid out at the start of this chapter?

The problem arises when your fears are unchecked or unsurrendered. While God designed fear as a protective mechanism, the enemy can manipulate your fears to keep you in bondage. Additionally, you may have developed limiting beliefs that trap you in repetitive cycles. To break free from these constraints, it's essential to cultivate awareness of your fears and continually submit them to God's guidance. This chapter will shed light on the constructive aspects of fear and the importance of managing it wisely.

Think of fear as your internal smoke detector. In and of themselves, smoke alarms are incredible inventions. They save lives and alert us of pending danger, but if it's misfiring or faulty as in the case of your fears sometimes, the consequences could be severe. The results can be fatal in the event of a real fire and the detector fails to alert you. It can be annoying if there is no fire but the detector keeps getting triggered (often prompting us to disconnect them, and then they can no longer alert us to real danger).

We once lived in an apartment that had a very sensitive smoke detector. That was an adventure within itself. The slightest provocation, like making toast or boiling water, would set it off. Picture the chaos: a mad scramble to reach the detector, frantic fanning to cool it down, and at times, resorting to pulling out the battery. It was an exercise in frustration. Fear, like that oversensitive smoke detector, has its role in keeping us safe. However, when it misfires it becomes a nuisance, going off at the most inconvenient and inappropriate moments.

These misfired fears can make you anxious about things that aren't genuinely threatening. It could be as harmless as misinterpreting a stranger's glance as disdain or taking an unreturned phone call as a personal rejection.

In the context of weight release, your internal fear alarm can unconsciously activate due to past experiences with weight loss and negative events during your formative years when food became your go-to coping mechanism.

> **Fear, like that oversensitive smoke detector, has a role in keeping us safe. However, when it misfires it becomes a nuisance, going off at the most inconvenient and inappropriate moments.**

Imagine the impact of these past experiences: perhaps it was the relentless dieting that never seemed to lead to lasting results, the taunts and jeers from peers during your school years, the disappointing look from your mother as you struggled to fit into the dress she bought for you, or the emotional turmoil that followed a difficult breakup. All these moments have etched themselves into the fabric of your life, leaving lasting imprints on your soul. They have woven a complex tapestry of fears and anxieties around the subject of weight and health.

These deep-seated fears are often buried deep in your subconscious, silently influencing your behaviors, choices, and emotional responses. They operate in the background, shaping your relationship with food, exercise, your body, and even God. So every time you try to lose weight, these old fears resurface even when there is no genuine danger. The memory of past struggles, disappointments, or hurtful comments triggers a subconscious fear response that can undermine your efforts.

So, just like our sensitive smoke detector, your internal fear alarm goes off at the most inconvenient times, hindering your progress on your weight release journey. But here's the good news: by acknowledging these past experiences, bringing them into the light of awareness, and actively working on healing and reprogramming your responses, you can begin to dismantle the intricate web of fear that has held you back. While this transformation may take time, it's a journey worth undertaking. With patience, understanding, and the grace of God, you can recalibrate your internal fear system and regain control over your health and well-being.

As you traverse the complexity of your weight-releasing journey, you'll be constantly paying attention for when the fears try to arise. Rather than reacting defensively or self-sabotaging, try to approach these fears with love and compassion. See them as God's loving hand gently guiding you to face your fears with faith.

In the upcoming chapters, we'll explore some of the self-sabotaging behaviors that often emerge in response to these unresolved fears. Here, let's explore a few examples of past events that, when left unhealed, can trigger self-sabotage in your weight releasing journey.

If you were left alone as a very young child by your parents or caregivers, this experience may have sensitized your internal fear alarm to an unhealthy fear of abandonment.

If your parents frequently engaged in conflict or fights during your formative years, your internal fear alarm might be hyper-sensitive to confrontation or anger.

For those who were made to feel worthless or shamed as children, your internal fear alarm may be hyper-sensitive to success or failure.

If you experienced any form of abuse in your past, this trauma could have set your internal fear alarm to be hyper-sensitive to rejection, often accompanied by intense feelings of guilt and shame.

Growing up with parents who were hard to please might have triggered a fear of failure.

The pattern is clear: past events and experiences can trigger a hyper-sensitivity to core fears, and this plays a significant role in your weight-releasing journey. In the next chapter, we'll explore a more comprehensive list of these core fears and how fear impacts your path to releasing weight.

Fear and Weight-Releasing

Fear, as we've been exploring, is undeniably one of the enemy's most potent weapons to keep God's people in bondage. The adversary possesses a deep understanding of your fears, at times more than you may even recognize within yourself. Armed with this knowledge, he skillfully manipulates your fears by falsely triggering your natural fear response. Instead of fear acting as a protective mechanism to safeguard you from danger and harm, it now frequently hinders you from taking essential actions. Conversely, it can send you into hyper-drive, attempting to extinguish metaphorical fires that pose no immediate peril. Understanding this dynamic is key to breaking free from the clutches of fear and moving toward lasting transformation.

When you embark on a weight loss journey, fear often rears its head because it initiates an internal conflict between your conscious mind—which consists of thoughts you're aware of and is primarily logical—and your subconscious mind—which harbors thoughts you may not consciously recognize and is heavily emotional. This internal tug-of-war arises from the fact that your conscious reasoning aligns with the idea that losing weight is beneficial and healthy. However, your subconscious mind, driven by emotional associations, links weight loss with concepts like pain, deprivation, loss of control, and potential harm. This cognitive dissonance represents your mind's attempt to reconcile these two opposing thoughts: good or bad, right or wrong, pleasure or pain. In such conflicts, emotions tend to triumph over logic leading you to make choices that defy your better judgment, like indulging in non-nutritious foods despite knowing their detrimental effects.

Now let's take a moment to reflect on your relationship with food during your formative years. Were these associations positive or laden with mixed emotions? Did food serve as a means to keep you quiet, or was it consistently scarce in your life? What was the atmosphere like around your family's dinner table? Perhaps family meals were a rarity, and you never experienced the traditional setting of sitting together for dinner. Were you subjected to hurtful names due to your weight, or did your mother take you to Weight Watchers at a young age? Were you the last to be chosen for school teams, and did food become your primary source of comfort? It's crucial to understand that until you reconcile these complex relationships with food and your body, they will continue to act as triggers for your fear response, making your weight loss journey a challenging and emotionally-charged endeavor.

Growing up in Trinidad, my experiences with body image and food were deeply shaped by the influence of my aunt, who raised my sisters and me. I remember her comments which, in her view, might have come across as cute or harmless but had a lasting impact on my self-esteem and relationship with food. One recurring theme in her remarks was my legs, which she often referred to as "tree trunk legs". These comments, though seemingly innocuous, carried the power to instill self-doubt and self-consciousness in a young, impressionable mind.

Moreover, I remember often being called "greedy-guts"—a nickname that stung and lingered in my memory. It not only emphasized the idea of overindulgence but also created a sense of guilt and shame around eating. These labels, however well-intentioned or playful they may have seemed at the time, laid the groundwork for a complicated relationship with my body and food.

In retrospect, these comments became part of the emotional baggage I carried into adulthood, affecting my perception of self-worth and contributing to a fear-based approach to food and weight management. The memory of those early experiences with body-shaming and food-related nicknames continued to be a driving force behind my struggles with weight and body image—even when I was at a seemingly ideal weight. Understanding and healing these emotional wounds were essential steps in my journey towards a healthier, more balanced relationship with food and a positive body image. It serves as a reminder of the power that early experiences and words can have in shaping our attitudes and behaviors in adulthood.

Understanding the profound impact of early experiences and core fears on your relationship with weight and food is crucial. It's akin to the invisible hand that guides your actions, often without your conscious awareness. You might be diligently trying to release weight, but your body's natural survival instincts are working against you, trying to protect you from perceived danger. In this case, the act of losing weight.

With this foundation in place, it's time to connect the dots between these core fears and your weight releasing journey. These fears, which often reside in your subconscious, can surface as formidable barriers when you commit to releasing weight. They come to the forefront of your mind, each carrying its own set of limiting beliefs that further complicate the process. Let's delve into some of the most relevant fears associated with weight loss, shedding light on the limiting beliefs that often accompany them:

1. Rejection: "Others won't accept the new me."

2. Failure: "What if I can't do it?"

3. Judgment: "What will others think?" "What new crazy thing is she trying now?" "She can't do it."

4. Feeling unwanted: "Food is my only friend."

5. Loneliness: "I'm all alone in this, no one else understands my struggle; I won't be able to do 'normal things.'"

6. Injury: "What if I hurt myself?"

7. Neglect: "No one cares about me."

8. Death: "I need food! What if I starve?"

9. Abandonment: "My husband/friends will leave me if I change."

10. Success: "Will I be able to maintain it? It's too much responsibility." "I'll attract the wrong attention."

11. Condemnation: "You're too vain." "I knew you would fail." "What's wrong with me?"

12. Humiliation: "I know what people are thinking about me when they see me." "I don't want to face them." "What if I lose the weight, only to regain it again?"

13. Losing Control: "What if I become obsessive?" "What if I can't control myself?"

14. Powerlessness: "What if I can't stop eating?" "Food is the only thing I can control." "I can't change."

15. Being misunderstood: "People will think…"

16. Rejection: "I'm not worth the time/investment." "Other people's needs are more important than mine."

Chances are, when you make an effort to lose weight one or more of these fears tend to arise within you, acting as formidable obstacles. The intensity of these (perceived) fears can be overwhelming, pushing you back into familiar patterns. Since most of them operate beneath your conscious awareness, you might not fully comprehend why you find yourself repeatedly self-sabotaging, making the same mistakes without a clear understanding of the underlying reasons.

As you continue on this journey, I'd like to share an open letter from one of our program graduates. It eloquently encapsulates the struggles and experiences that many of our clients face. By the end of this chapter, my hope is that you will also discover the liberation that comes from learning how to reframe your fears and gain mastery over them.

> Dear Fear,
>
> I've seen you steal from me. I've seen you ravage my life, robbing me of joy, connection, feeling competent, feeling adequate, of knowing myself, and knowing my Creator.
>
> You succeeded for a while at cutting me off from Him almost completely, flooding my mind with thoughts revolving around me… Keeping me chasing my own tail in an exhausting exercise in futility.
>
> Like a rampant cancer, the self-centered fear devoured me. It took over my mind. It was the driving force in my life. "How do I protect myself from being exposed? How do I hide that I don't have all the answers?" I would ask myself. You had me chasing things, people, and feelings that would protect me from the shame of my human imper-

fection. I have borne these dark secrets as a weighty yoke, dragging me around and down by the neck.

You made me afraid to try, to fail, to succeed, to be wrong, to shine, to stand, to be broken, empty, and weak. You made me ashamed to be human. Then, you used your evil cousins Pride and Perfectionism to further cut me off from the loving, Almighty God who created me.

You enticed me to hide behind their smokescreen, right where you wanted me, you evil liar!! You wanted me behind that smoke so when I looked out, things seemed fuzzy and blurry. So that your evil companions of Doubt and Insecurity could handcuff me to the prison of myself; where the light of my God, who came for me in the form of Jesus Christ, looked so far from me.

You deceived me, you lying thief! You had me right where you wanted me, believing your lies, terrified to take the very chances that would bring me freedom!

Well done, I'll give you that! But I'm here to say that it's over!!! You cannot have me anymore! I belong to Jesus Christ and claim victory through His blood over you, Satan, and every single one of your lousy, evil minions and over each one of your spirit slaves who bow down to you in the fiery pit of hell.

I will not bow down to you like they do! My Lord, my God, my Creator, my Vindicator, my Savior, my Redeemer, my Protector, Jesus Christ is the only one I will ever bow to. I am His and His alone. He owns me. He's the author of me, and as such, has the only authority over me and my life. I will subject every part of me to Him. You can't touch me now!

So, Fear, I won't be needing you anymore! I'm taking off your iron yoke of slavery and springing free of the shackles that I've grown so accustomed to.

Instead, I'm taking up His yoke which is easy, and the burden light. You may try to come against me, but know that by the blood of Jesus Christ, my Savior, you will never again prosper over me!

Go back to hell where you came from!!

His humble child,

Geri

Fear in the Bible: Abraham's Experience

Abraham, often regarded as the father of the nations, provides us with valuable insights into the dynamics of fear and how it keep us from embracing all God has for us. God made remarkable promises to Abraham, then known as Abram:

"I will make you a great nation; I will bless you and make your name great; and you shall be a blessing. I will bless those who bless you, and I will curse him who curses you; and in you, all the families of the earth shall be blessed" (Genesis 12:2-3 NIV).

These promises were truly extraordinary, yet we witness Abraham's recurrent struggles with fear. He makes numerous decisions based on fear and doubt, leading him down the wrong path.

It's not hard to empathize with Abraham's struggle with fear and doubt. After all, he had several reasons to doubt God repeatedly. God had promised to provide him with land, and it fell prey to famine (Genesis 12:10). Despite the assurance of numerous children, he remained childless well into his advanced years (Genesis 15:2).

Abraham's fear-driven decisions led him to deception on several occasions. Twice, he claimed that his wife, Sarai (later Sarah), was his sister (Genesis 12:11-13; 20:1-2,5) in situations where he believed his life was in danger. He also resorted to sleeping with his Egyptian servant, Hagar, in an attempt to fulfill God's promise of offspring (Genesis 16:4). This illustrates the human tendency to take matters into our own hands when we perceive that circumstances are not unfolding in our favor. Abraham's actions were driven by fear and a desire to ensure his own safety and legacy, even when it meant compromising God's promises. Can you relate?

Despite Abraham's fears sometimes getting the best of him, God consistently intervened to protect him. In Genesis 12:17, "the Lord plagued Pharaoh and his house with great plagues because of Sarai, Abram's wife."

In Genesis 15, Abraham is once again gripped by fear. After defeating his enemies (Genesis 14:17), he is now living in fear for his life. In response, God addresses Abraham's fears directly, addressing his deepest core fear—the lack of a legacy (children).

Abraham needed to feel safe, accomplished, and assured that his legacy would extend beyond him. God speaks directly to these needs by declaring Himself as Abraham's provider and protector and by giving him a vision. God assures him that his reward will be great (Genesis 15:1). Despite the importance of these needs, God recognized Abraham's deepest core fear of lacking a legacy (children) and addressed it:

"Abram said, 'God, Master, what use are your gifts as long as I'm childless and Eliezer of Damascus is going to inherit everything?' Abram continued, 'See, you've given me no children, and now a mere house servant is going to get it all'" (Genesis 15:2-3).

In response, God reassures Abraham: "This man will not be your heir, but a son who is your own flesh and blood will be your heir" (Genesis 15:4).

As time passes, Abraham's faith steadily grows. The ultimate test arrives when God asks him to sacrifice his only son (Genesis 22:2). Whether he still experiences fear at this point becomes irrelevant. God has fortified his character and deepened his capacity to obey to the extent that he would unquestioningly act on whatever God instructed him to do. As a result, Abraham reaps abundant blessings (Genesis 23:15-18).

God used Abraham's doubts and fears as building blocks for faith, fortifying his character and teaching him to trust and learn from God. Similarly, you bear the responsibility to confront your fears, not run from them, and use them as an opportunity to cast your cares onto your Heavenly Father. If you don't break the cycle of letting your fears control you, you risk passing them on to your children. In later generations, Isaac, Abraham's son, repeats the same pattern and lies about his wife, Rebekah, being his sister (Genesis 26:7). Sadly, the pattern of fear-induced behaviors doesn't stop with Isaac. It extends to the next generation as well. Isaac's sons, particularly Joseph's brothers, allowed their fear and envy to lead them to deceive their father and sell their brother Joseph into slavery. The intergenerational transmission of fear-driven behaviors is why we must address these core fears. Otherwise, they will continue to shape family dynamics and lead to destructive actions that affect the well-being of family members and individuals.

Throughout the Bible, we see how God transforms people from fear-driven lives to faith-filled ones, and He will do it for you, too. Like Abraham, your fears may appear insurmountable, making it seem impossible to believe in God's promises when you've faced disappointment numerous times and it feels like you'll never achieve your goal. Yet, take heart; you're on a journey which will take you back to the heart of God. Through this reconnection, you'll learn how to stand on God's promises and live in faith rather than fear. This transformation will make all the difference in your weight releasing journey.

How to Identify Your Physiological Response to Fear

The challenge with identifying your core fears is that they are subconscious. You're rarely aware of what triggered them. One minute you can be laughing hysterically at a joke and the next minute you can feel your heart racing and palms sweating because of a seemingly random interaction with someone. Thankfully, sensations in your physical body can give us some insight into what's going on in our minds and spirit.

As a tripartite being, you exist in a body, possess a soul, and are a spirit, as referenced in passages like 1 Thessalonians 5:23 and Hebrews 4:12. Your physical body serves as the outer shell housing the temple of the living God, as noted in 1 Corinthians 6:19-20. This body acts as the outward expression of what's transpiring in your soul, similar to how a nervous tic or rapid speech can indicate inner turmoil. Overeating, too, can be a symptom of an underlying internal issue.

The beauty of this understanding is that even if you're not immediately conscious of what triggered your specific fear, you can identify your physical response to it. Recognizing this response places you in a position to work backward and uncover the underlying trigger. So, while you might not be able to name the precise fear, your body's physiological response serves as an alert, signaling that something is amiss.

However, if you continuously address only the symptoms without delving into the root causes of why you overeat, you'll find yourself perpetually on another diet attempting to treat the effects (excess weight) rather than addressing the cause (fear). In essence, excess weight is a symptom, not the root issue. To assist you in identifying when your fear response has been triggered, here are various physiological indicators, ranging from mild to severe, that your body employs as warning signals, indicating the need for attention:

- Increased heart rate
- A sinking feeling in the pit of your stomach
- A lump-like sensation in your throat
- Sweaty palms
- Nervous laughter
- Anger
- Urge to run
- Urge to hide
- Urge to eat
- Dry mouth
- Alterations in your voice, potentially speaking in a higher pitch or experiencing stuttering
- An increase in body temperature
- Flushing of the face
- Becoming unusually talkative or clamming up
- Excessive smiling
- Extra politeness
- Racing thoughts
- Voice cracking
- Trembling
- Nausea

- General anxiety or panic attacks
- Feeling light-headed or dizzy
- Loosening of bowels
- Goosebumps
- Freezing up
- Cravings to eat, drink, or engage in pacifying behaviors

As you develop an awareness of how these fear responses manifest in your body, you empower yourself to take meaningful action.

Applying the 3-Step Reset to Fear

Up to this point, you've harnessed the power of the 3-Step Reset to achieve a calm nervous system and reduce stress, employed it to overcome eating challenges, and even applied it to master your morning routine. Now, you're about to uncover how this tool can be used to transform your fear into faith. This technique has proven its effectiveness in various aspects of your journey, and will continue to serve as a valuable resource to help you silence that fire alarm that's constantly misfiring in your mind and often triggering you to overeat or make unhealthy choices that don't serve your highest self.

As you now recognize, your core fears are ground zero for your internal turmoil; your unhealthy relationship with food, exercise, and your body. Like records playing over and over in your head, they are ingrained within your subconscious mind and taint your beliefs about yourself, the world, and God.

You've also identified that when your core fears are triggered, your immediate instinct is to stop the pain. Instinctively and rightfully so, you want to avoid this pain at all costs. No one wants to feel pain, so you avoid it with distractions like TV, the internet, people, shopping, and food.

But you can probably attest that this relief is only temporary, and as soon as your fear button is pushed again you react the exact same way. There is nothing on this Earth that can take away that pain but God.

Step 1: Pause

When you encounter fear it's important to identify it by being attuned to your physiological responses, as listed in the previous chapter. Pause and take a deep breath. Instead of succumbing to the control or overwhelming nature of fear, this step encourages you to embrace and sit with the discomfort without an immediate reaction.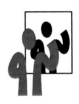

In that moment, reframe your perspective on fear. Recognize it as a signal that something in your life requires your attention. This is your opportunity to acknowledge fear and invite God into the situation. Embrace fear with gratitude, love, and compassion, expressing thanks for making you aware that something in your spirit, soul, or body needs attention. By pausing and responding in this way, you begin to transform your relationship with fear, turning it from an obstacle into a catalyst for positive change.

Imagine you're faced with a challenging situation that triggers fear. Your heart starts racing and you feel a knot in your stomach. Your first response might be to stuff the feeling with food. Instead of immediately reacting with anxiety or panic and suppressing the feeling, you remain still. You pause and take a deep breath. In that moment, you sit with the discomfort and acknowledge your fear.

As you do this, you reframe your perspective on fear. You see it as a signal, a message from within, telling you that something is out of alignment. The power of the pause will allow your internal fire alarm called fear to be used for its intended purpose, which is to lead you to safety.

Step 2: Pray

Once you've paused to calm your nervous system and avoid impulsive reactions, it's time to surrender your fear to God and invite Him to fulfill the deeper need within you. Remember, all fears can be viewed as needs that only God can truly satisfy.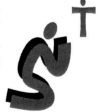

Here's how you can approach this step:

1. Look at the list of fears and the corresponding wants or needs that you require God to fulfill:

- Fear: Rejection ➲ Want/Need: Acceptance and Trust

- Fear: Failure ➲ Want/Need: Success

- Fear: Judgment ➲ Want/Need: Grace and Unconditional Love

- Fear: Feeling Unwanted ➲ Want/Need: Love and Acceptance

- Fear: Loneliness ➲ Want/Need: Companionship

- Fear: Injury ➲ Want/Need: Safety

- Fear: Neglect ➲ Want/Need: Love and Affirmation

- Fear: Death ➲ Want/Need: Life and Vitality

- Fear: Abandonment ➲ Want/Need: Support and Affirmation

- Fear: Success ➲ Want/Need: Affirmation, Ongoing Support, and Unconditional Love

- Fear: Condemnation ➲ Want/Need: Acceptance

- Fear: Humiliation ➲ Want/Need: Edification and Grace

- Fear: Losing Control ➲ Want/Need: Calm and Peace

- Fear: Inferiority ➲ Want/Need: Self-esteem and Affirmation

- Fear: Powerlessness ➲ Want/Need: Courage, Strength, and Hope

- Fear: Being Misunderstood ➲ Want/Need: Acknowledgment, Acceptance, and Grace

- Fear: Feeling Worthless ➲ Want/Need: Self-esteem and Love

- Fear: Feeling Devalued ➲ Want/Need: Value and Acceptance

Here's an example of what this could look like:

> You've been working on a project at your workplace, and it's finally time for the team to present their findings to the higher-ups. During the presentation, you share your ideas confidently, but as the meeting progresses you notice some of your colleagues making dismissive comments or showing disinterest in your contributions. After

the meeting, you hear that your suggestions were not included in the final plan.

You feel those familiar feelings of rejection well up in you and all you can think about is stopping at your favorite drive-through to feel better. Instead, reframe that feeling of rejection and invite God to fill your need for affirmation and validation from Him. Your prayer could go like this:

"Dear God, today in that meeting, I felt like a door slamming shut in my face. It stung to watch my ideas crumble, ignored and brushed aside. But I'm clinging to the knowledge that in You there's acceptance and trust waiting for me. This feeling is heavy on my chest, and I lay it at Your feet. Please fill my heart with Your rock-solid acceptance, and help me rest in Your love. I'm shouting from the depths of my soul: I am accepted in Your eyes, and I'm anchoring myself in Your unwavering love. Rejection at work may bruise, but it won't break me because I'm held tight in Your embrace. You're my sanctuary, my refuge, and my unshakeable strength. In Your presence, I find the solace of being wholly accepted and cherished. Amen."

With practice, you'll become more adept at recognizing fear as an alert to unmet core needs. Thank fear for its role in highlighting these needs, and then turn your fears over to God, allowing Him to fill these unmet needs and wants.

Commit to fervent prayer, asking God to fill these needs every time you feel fear. Follow the example of David in Psalms 139:23, asking God to search your fearful and anxious thoughts. This is the quickest way to reframe your fears, transforming them into opportunities for God to provide.

Step 3: (Active) Practice for Fear

In this Active Practice for fear of rejection, you will create a physical movement to establish a positive association with the fear you're addressing. By repeating this action, you can rewire your thought patterns and responses, gradually replacing fear with faith and trust. Here's how to perform this Active Practice: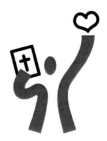

Choose Your Physical Action: Select a simple physical movement that resonates with you and symbolizes God's love, acceptance, and protection. This movement should provide a sense of comfort and safety. For example, you can choose to give yourself a warm hug, gently placing your hands on your heart, or clasping your hands in a reassuring manner.

Over time, you can be proactive and recognize situations or moments when your fear is likely to arise. It could be during a challenging meeting, a social event, or when facing potential rejection. Be mindful of these triggers and remember to use your Active Practice when necessary.

As you actively engage in this transformative process, you will find that your fear of rejection, or any other fear you're addressing, no longer wields the same power over you. You are rewiring your thought patterns and emotional responses, replacing fear with faith and trust in God's love and acceptance.

Imagine a future where, in a challenging meeting, a tense conversation, when faced with a daunting task, or as you try something new, your heart no longer races with fear, and the urge to seek solace in food no longer haunts you. Instead of allowing fear to take hold, you've learned to pause, take a deep breath, and initiate your chosen physical action.

This three-step process empowers you to acknowledge and address your fears, turning them into catalysts for positive change. You are no longer controlled by fear; you have the tools to invite God into your fears, trusting in His love and protection. As you continue to practice these steps, you will find the strength to face your fears with faith, knowing that you are accepted, valued, and cherished in His presence.

Principle 12 Summary

Reflect on these key points:

- Self-sabotage is a familiar companion, often driven by underlying fears that can be addressed and transformed.

- The very nature of trying to lose weight triggers resistance and unleashes a cascade of emotions that can lead to self-sabotage.

- The 3-Step Reset is a powerful tool to keep your core fears from sabotaging you.

Principle #13: Develop Mental Resiliency

Master Your Mind

In the last chapter you discovered that fear is at the root of why you've been perpetually self-sabotaging your weight releasing efforts. We briefly journeyed to the Garden of Eden to understand the origin of fear. We recognized that prior to the fall, Adam walked freely in perfect fellowship with God. But after the fall, sin entered the world and with it it's companion, fear. In this chapter, you will gain deeper understanding how your core fears have given rise to limiting beliefs that reinforce your fears, creating a cycle that can feel inescapable. As you learned to uproot the core fears, you'll also learn how to identify and pluck up limiting beliefs that sabotage your health and weight releasing efforts.

As I pen these words, I find myself in a personal journey of quieting my ever-racing mind, a journey that was set in motion by a deep revelation during my prayer time a couple of months ago. It was a moment of divine communication that left a lasting impact on my understanding of the inner workings of the mind.

In that sacred moment, I heard the Lord's gentle whisper, "You've surrendered your daily life to me, but there's a whole other world that you're living in your head, and there's a whole lot more going on in there. I want that life, too." The weight of those words struck me like a revelation I had never before considered. I had never thought of the thoughts in my head as having a life of their own. In essence, my mind was a realm unto itself, with thoughts, emotions, and a constant whirlwind of activity. It was no wonder

I often found myself living with a low-level anxiety, a background noise that I had grown accustomed to.

So, in response to this heart-to-heart moment with God, I felt led to fast from all forms of social media. It was a deliberate choice to disengage from the digital world temporarily, to step away from the constant influx of information and the never-ending scroll of curated content. This decision allowed me to confront the intricate web of thoughts and distractions that had taken root in my mind.

Romans 8:6 says that "The mind governed by the flesh is death, but the mind governed by the Spirit is life and peace." This is how I define mental resilience. It's the ability to cultivate a mindset that aligns with the principles and guidance of the Holy Spirit. It's the ability to persevere in spite of the negative influences of worldly distractions, temptations, self-doubt and limiting beliefs, which can lead to spiritual and emotional death.

Conversely, the "mind governed by the Spirit" signifies a state of alignment and union with God where thoughts are guided by a deeper wisdom, purpose, and calling. It's a mind that seeks life, freedom, joy, and peace.

In the chapters that follow, you will discover how to develop mental resilience. Now, you might wonder how this relates to your health and weight loss journey. When your mind is cluttered with distractions and comparisons, it can lead to stress, emotional eating, and a sense of disconnection from your true self. Also, it's your mind that tells your body what to do. You thought about dessert long before it found its way into your mouth. When you learn how to take every thought captive as 2 Cor. 10:5 teaches us, you can stop those cravings from sabotaging you. A popular quote captures the essence of this scripture: "No thought lives in your head rent-free."

As you develop mental resilience, you learn how to reframe your limiting beliefs and regain control over your thoughts, steering them toward your health and weight loss goals. My hope is that understanding that no thought lives in your head rent-free empowers you to choose which thoughts to nurture and which to cast aside, which thoughts are worth the investment, and which ones are squatting on the valuable real-estate in your mind.

God's Word gives us the template for how we are to do that. It's found in one of my favorite scriptures, Romans 12:2 (ESV).

"Do not be conformed to this world, but be transformed by the renewal of your mind, that by testing you may discern what is the will of God, what is good and acceptable and perfect."

The author, Paul, wrote the Epistle to the Romans to the Christian community in Rome. In this letter, he addressed various theological and practical aspects of the Christian faith. In Romans 12, Paul shifts his focus to practical instructions for Christian living. He encourages believers to live in a way that reflects their faith and to present their bodies as living sacrifices to God.

In Romans 12:2, Paul emphasizes the importance of not conforming to the patterns of the world but instead being transformed by the renewal of one's mind. The context here is about the transformation of a believer's life through faith in Christ and the indwelling of the Holy Spirit. Paul is urging Christians to have a renewed mindset, one that aligns with God's will and is characterized by moral and spiritual transformation.

The reason he is saying this is to highlight the importance of aligning one's life with God's will. Paul is instructing believers to move away from the worldly mindset and behaviors that characterized their lives before coming to faith in Christ. By renewing their minds and living according to God's will, they would experience spiritual growth and transformation.

Paul is calling for a change in thinking and living that reflects the Christian faith, where believers are not conformed to the values and behaviors of the surrounding culture but instead are being transformed into the likeness of Christ through the renewal of their minds. This transformation is seen as a response to God's mercy and a way to live a life that is pleasing to Him.

The concept of a "conformed mind" is in stark contrast to a "transformed mind". A conformed mind is shaped by the values and norms of the world, often prioritizing material gain, following societal trends unquestioningly, and lacking discernment. In contrast, a transformed mind is deeply influenced by God's Word, prioritizes spiritual growth and love for others, actively renews its thinking with Biblical truths, and exercises discernment in all aspects of life. This distinction emphasizes the importance of aligning one's thinking with God's will and experiencing spiritual transformation rather than conforming to worldly patterns.

Here is my interpretation of the contrast that Paul makes between a conformed and transformed mind as it relates to your health journey:

A transformed mind makes choices that honor God by nourishing your body with wholesome foods, engaging in regular physical activity, and managing stress in healthy ways. Your motivation for weight release is rooted in a desire to glorify God through a healthier lifestyle, stewarding your temple, and seeing yourself as God sees you. This mind stands firm in God's promises and truths.

A conformed mind makes choices influenced by external pressures or societal expectations, leading to a focus on short-term results rather than long-term well-being. This can result in unsustainable weight loss methods or cycles of dieting and overindulging. This mind is focused on failure, what it can't do, mistakes of the past, and poor self-perception.

This distinction between a conformed mind and a transformed mind will be important going forward because we want to keep living from our conformed mind as we reject the thoughts that flow from our transformed mind.

In the last chapter, I used the analogy of a faulty smoke detector to explain how our core fear keeps us on high alert and anxious. Just as the alarm sound is meant to protect you from danger, your core fears are there to safeguard you from perceived threats. However, when the smoke detector becomes too sensitive, it triggers false alarms even when there's no real danger. This results in unnecessary panic and disruption.

Let's stay with that analogy to discuss limiting beliefs and how they keep you perpetuating a set of feelings like self-doubt, discouragement, despair, and defeat in your weight releasing journey. If your core fear is the oversensitive smoke detector or fire alarm, limiting beliefs are the faulty wiring that keeps tripping the smoke detector. Imagine limiting beliefs as the faulty wiring within your thought patterns. They have the potential to cause your core fears to activate needlessly or in response to situations that don't merit such a strong reaction. For example, if you hold a limiting belief that you're unworthy of love or success, this belief can lead to your core fear of rejection or failure being triggered even in situations where there's no actual threat.

Much like the smoke detector or fire alarm can generate false alarms that disrupt your daily life, limiting beliefs can produce false alarms within your mind. These false alarms may result in self-sabotage when it comes to managing your weight. For instance, if you believe that you're destined to be overweight and incapable of change, this belief can become a self-fulfilling prophecy. It may deter you from fully committing to a healthy lifestyle because you've convinced yourself that it won't make a difference. Another limiting belief you may have is the notion that your worth is determined solely by your physical appearance. This harmful belief can lead to unhealthy relationships with food, body image and self-esteem, again hindering your weight management efforts. The interplay between core fears and limiting beliefs can leave you trapped in a cycle of yo-yo dieting, where progress feels elusive. However, by developing a deeper understanding of these limiting beliefs and the role they play in your life, you can begin to break free from this cycle and move towards a more compassionate and empowered relationship with yourself and your weight management journey.

Understanding Limiting Beliefs

What if someone asked you if you believe you will ever achieve your goal? How might you have responded in the past? Your answer is a good starting point for introspection and self-examination, allowing you to identify and confront the limiting beliefs that may be holding you back from your health and weight management journey.

As you explore this, consider some common limiting beliefs that may have crossed your mind, such as:

1. "No, because I have a slow metabolism."

2. "I was born this way."

3. "I can't do it; it's too hard."

4. "I have too much weight to lose."

5. "It's my genetics."

6. "My injury/limitation/illness keeps me from doing what I want to."

7. "Nothing works, it doesn't matter what I do."

8. "I hate exercise."

9. "I don't like any of the foods that will help me lose weight."

10. "I will only put the weight back on anyway."

These are just a few examples of the limiting beliefs that can hinder your progress in achieving your health and weight management goals. This chapter will guide you on a journey to recognize, confront, and reframe these limiting beliefs.

In our fallen world, we provide ourselves with an endless supply of reasons that we will not succeed. If you're not aware, they will crush you under their snare if you're not vigilant in weeding them out of your thoughts, your vocabulary, and your actions.

Limiting beliefs are engrained thoughts, thinking patterns, or beliefs that we hold about ourselves and our world. They are one of the many reasons we struggle with our weight.

These beliefs or positions about life are self-limiting, and that's what makes them so deadly. As we unconsciously carry these beliefs with us into adulthood, they often sabotage our plans and goals, and most importantly God's best for us.

Limiting beliefs, deeply ingrained in our minds and hearts, act as the silent architects of our self-sabotaging behaviors and emotional struggles. They are the underlying causes of several detrimental patterns that hinder our progress on the journey to better health and weight management.

1. Procrastination. Limiting beliefs often whisper in our minds, convincing us that we're not capable or that success is unattainable. This internal dialogue of doubt and negativity leads to procrastination. We delay taking action because these beliefs make us question whether our efforts are worth it.

2. Blame. When we harbor limiting beliefs, it becomes easier to point fingers at external factors or other people for our challenges. These beliefs can make us think that we're not responsible for our actions or outcomes, shifting blame away from ourselves.

3. Excuses. Limiting beliefs provide a ready arsenal of excuses. They tell

us that we can't do something because we're too old, not talented enough, or that our circumstances are insurmountable. This results in a cycle of making excuses instead of taking initiative.

4. Low Self-esteem. These beliefs have a way of eroding our self-worth. They make us question our abilities and value, leading to low self-esteem. A healthy sense of self-worth is crucial for the confidence and motivation needed to make positive changes.

5. Emotional Eating. Emotional eating as we discussed in previous chapters is often a response to stress, anxiety, or other emotions. Limiting beliefs can amplify these emotions and drive us to seek comfort in food.

If we hold on to these beliefs, they will negatively taint our view about who we are, what we can do, and/or who God is. They will keep us from fully and properly seeking after God.

In this chapter, we'll confront and conquer these limiting beliefs, clearing the path to mental resilience.

Let's look at an example in the Bible to see the impact of limited beliefs.

Limiting beliefs are powerfully illustrated through the Biblical story of Joshua and Caleb versus the ten spies. This story comes from the Book of Numbers in the Old Testament. The Israelites, led by Moses, had been delivered from slavery in Egypt and were on the cusp of entering the Promised Land. Moses sent twelve spies, one from each tribe, to scout the land of Canaan.

Upon their return, the spies' reports were divided into two groups. Joshua and Caleb, representing one group, brought back an optimistic and faith-filled account of the land. They described it as a bountiful and fruitful land that God had promised to give them. Their focus was on the possibility, the promise, and the power of God.

However, the other ten spies painted a very different picture. They focused on the challenges and obstacles they saw, emphasizing the giants and the fortified cities. Their report was filled with fear and doubt, highlighting their limiting beliefs about their ability to conquer the land.

The stark contrast between these two perspectives reflects the power of limiting beliefs. Joshua and Caleb had faith in God's promise and His ability to help them overcome any obstacle. They saw themselves as capable and empowered by God to fulfill His plan. On the other hand, the ten spies allowed their fears and self-doubt to shape their perception of the situation. Their limiting beliefs hindered them from embracing the promise and moving forward with faith.

In the end, the Israelites as a whole chose to listen to the ten spies, leading to forty years of wandering in the wilderness. Joshua and Caleb, the minority with unwavering faith, were the only two from their generation who eventually entered the Promised Land.

Refuse to let your limiting beliefs prevent you from stepping into the fullness of God's plan for your life. The story is a powerful reminder that your beliefs about your capabilities, along with your trust in God's promises, can have a lasting impact on the course of our journey. Just as Joshua and Caleb held to their faith and overcame the giants, you can break free from limiting beliefs and move toward the abundant life that God intends for us.

Three Types of Limiting Beliefs

When it comes to weight releasing, your limiting beliefs can be identified in one of three categories. The result is always the same. They keep you from achieving your goals and keep you from achieving all that God has for you. Let's look at each of them individually.

Limiting Beliefs About Yourself

Firstly, you encounter limiting beliefs about yourself. These deep-rooted assumptions regarding your own abilities, talents, or resources can have a great impact on your success. They creep into your thoughts with phrases such as:

- I'm too old for this.
- I can't help it, I'm just big-boned.
- I'm the world's biggest procrastinator.
- I guess I just don't have the willpower.
- I'm a quitter. I never finish what I start.

Limiting Beliefs About People

Secondly, limiting beliefs can extend to your perceptions of other people or the world at large. These beliefs may lead you to believe that external factors, or even the actions of others, are insurmountable obstacles to your success. They manifest in thoughts like:

- Why bother? They won't listen to me anyway.
- What does she know?
- They're too advanced for me.
- She's too overweight to be a marathon runner.
- She hasn't responded, I guess she's mad at me.
- Overweight people have slow metabolisms.
- Wanting to be an ideal weight is vanity.
- You can't successfully lose weight without restricting your calories.

Limiting Beliefs About God and Faith

Lastly, limiting beliefs can infiltrate your spiritual life, affecting your relationship with God and faith. These beliefs may restrict your willingness to approach God or distort your understanding of His limitless power and grace. You might find yourself thinking:

- I can't keep sinning and going to God.
- God knows my heart, so I don't need to tell Him what He already knows.
- God cannot bless my mess.
- If I'm a Christian then I should...
- If only I had more faith, then God would answer my prayers.
- If God is so powerful, then…

Now that you have a clearer understanding of the types of limiting beliefs, let's explore their connections with the core fears discussed in previous chapters. The list of limiting beliefs on the right is closely linked to specific fears on the left. Addressing your root fear can help you confront these limiting beliefs, and challenging the limiting beliefs can help you overcome your core fears. It's not a choice between one or the other; it's a simultaneous process of addressing both.

Limiting Beliefs:

1. "Others won't accept the new me." - Fear: Rejection

2. "I can't do it." - Fear: Failure

3. "What will others think? "What new crazy thing is she trying now?" "It's just a matter of time before she fails again." - Fear: Judgment

4. "Food is my only friend." - Fear: Feeling unwanted

5. "I'm all alone in this, no one else understands my struggle; I won't be able to do 'normal things'." - Fear: Loneliness

6. "What if I hurt myself?" - Fear: Injury

7. "No one cares about me." - Fear: Neglect

8. "I need food! What if I starve?" - Fear: Death

9. "My husband/friends will leave me if I change." - Fear: Abandonment

10. "I won't be able to maintain it. It's too much responsibility." "I'll attract the wrong attention." - Fear: Success

11. "You're too vain." "I knew you would fail." "What's wrong with me?" - Fear: Condemnation

12. "I know what people are thinking about me when they see me." "I don't want to face them." "What if I lose the weight, only to regain it - again?" - Fear: Humiliation

13. "What if I become obsessive?" "What if I can't control myself?" - Fear: Losing control

14. "What if I can't stop eating?" "Food is the only thing I can control." "I can't change." - Fear: Powerlessness

15. "People will think..." - Fear: Being misunderstood

16. "I'm not worth the time/investment." "Other people's needs are more important than mine." - Fear: Rejection

Can you relate to any of these limiting beliefs? Do you see how they may be hindering you from experiencing all that God has in store for you? Confronting and dismantling these beliefs is a crucial step in your journey to release weight and embrace God's plan for your life.

Let's summarize by going back to our faulty smoke detector. Your limiting beliefs are like the flawed connections that trigger the fear response, much like the malfunctioning wiring in a smoke detector can set off false alarms. Just as the faulty wiring in a smoke detector can lead to unnecessary alarms, the limiting beliefs act as the faulty wiring in your thought processes, causing unnecessary fear responses in your weight and health journey. This fear response can lead to stress, emotional eating, and self-sabotage.

Let's go to our 3-Step Reset once again to address your limiting beliefs. They are key to helping you develop emotional resilience.

Step 1: Pause

The pause will be critical in helping you overcome limiting beliefs. Although this pause will serve once again to calm your nervous system, it serves another purpose: to bring you into the present moment. You see, limiting beliefs pull you into the past and try to keep you anchored there. However, God is here in the present, waiting for you to fully embrace the now.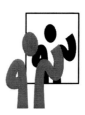

In this moment of pause, you have the opportunity to release the grip of limiting beliefs that are tied to past experiences or future anxieties. By grounding yourself in the present, you can release everything to God and allow Him to meet you in real time. This step allows you to let go of the baggage from the past and the worries about the future, creating space for mental resilience to grow and flourish.

Not only are limiting beliefs often rooted in past events or future anxieties, but they are also subconscious. That's why pausing is crucial; it allows us to move them from the subconscious to our conscious mind. This process of bringing them into the light of your consciousness is essential to confront and ultimately overcome these beliefs that have held you back for so long.

By pausing and becoming aware of these limiting beliefs, you start to shine a light on the hidden corners of your mind where they dwell. When you consciously acknowledge them, you gain the power to challenge and replace them with God's transformative truth. This is akin to rewiring your mental circuitry. Just as a faulty smoke detector needs to be identified and replaced with a working one, your limiting beliefs must be recognized and replaced with the truth of God's Word. That's Step 2.

As you take that critical pause, it allows you to gain a clearer perspective on the lies that these limiting beliefs represent. It's as though the enemy was attempting to deceive you, but in that moment of pause you see through the trickery. It's like shining a light on the darkness of your thoughts and realizing that what you once believed to be insurmountable barriers were, in fact, deceptive illusions. This heightened awareness enables you to discern the falsehoods and recognize them for what they are: attempts to hinder your progress and keep you from experiencing the freedom and transformation that God has in store for you.

Last year, my mom underwent laser eye surgery. She had struggled with her vision for years, and the surgery was a long-awaited solution. What struck me most was her reaction after the procedure. She was absolutely amazed at the newfound clarity in her vision. The world that had once appeared hazy and indistinct suddenly came into sharp focus. It was like she had been given a fresh pair of eyes, and she marveled at the beauty of the world like never before.

That what the power of the "pause" will do in our journey to overcome limiting beliefs. Before the surgery my mom's vision was clouded by imperfections in her eyes, much like how limiting beliefs cloud our minds. These beliefs are like the distorted lenses through which we perceive ourselves, our capabilities, and our worth. They create a distorted reality that keeps us from reaching our full potential.

However, the pause brings things into focus. It allows you to see more clearly, just as the surgery did for my mom. During this pause, you gain a new perspective free from the fog of limiting beliefs. It's as if a veil is lifted, and you start to discern the lies and fears that were previously hidden.

This moment of clarity is invaluable. It enables you to confront and dismantle the illusions that have held you back. It's like a fresh pair of eyes, providing a sharper, more accurate view of your life, your potential, and your connection with God. The pause allows you to cast off the cloudy lenses of limiting beliefs, making way for a brighter, more fulfilling future.

Step 2: Pray

As you develop awareness of your limiting beliefs, you will begin to reframe your beliefs. Reframing is the process of changing the way you perceive and interpret a situation or belief. Reframing can be done through prayer, declaration, or simply through conscious self-talk. Here is a list of limiting beliefs that you can use declarations to reframe.

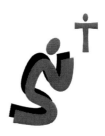

- I can't trust myself around certain foods.

- I am empowered to make wise choices and rely on God's strength to resist temptations.

- I love food too much to lose weight.

- I find satisfaction in nourishing my body and seek God's guidance to develop a healthy relationship with food.

- I can't stop eating food when it tastes really good.

- I honor my body as a temple of the Holy Spirit and practice self-control, enjoying food in moderation.

- It's not possible to lose weight after menopause.

- With God all things are possible, including achieving and maintaining a healthy weight at any stage of life.

- I can't lose weight because I have no willpower.

- I draw strength from God, Who strengthens me and enables me to make disciplined choices for my well-being.

If the same beliefs come up over and over, memorize one or more of these declarations, or put them in prominent places where you'll notice them.

Step 3: Active Practice

By now, hopefully you've got the hang of the Active Practice. As you make your declaration, select a simple physical movement that reinforces your confession. It could be the same one you've used throughout this book or it could be a new one that emphasizes the declaration. This movement should provide a sense of comfort and safety, gently placing your hands on your heart, or raising your hand in surrender.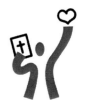

My friend, know that we have the tools to reset and rewire your thought processes for a brighter, more resilient future

The 3-Step Reset is your guide to developing mental resilience and overcoming limiting beliefs. Remember, you have the power to rewire your mental circuitry. As you practice the 3-Step Reset, you'll be well on your way to conquering limiting beliefs, developing mental resilience, and experiencing the freedom and transformation that God has in store for you on your weight and health journey. It's a journey toward embracing the now, seeing through the trickery of limiting beliefs, and finding a brighter, more fulfilling future.

Principle 13 Summary

Reflect on these key points:

- Recognize that limiting beliefs, often rooted in fear, can lead to self-sabotage in your weight release journey. They act like faulty wiring in your smoke detector, causing panic and disruption.

- Limiting beliefs fall into three categories: about yourself, about people, and about God and faith. They greatly affect your success and self-perception, hindering your path to better health.

- Challenge and confront these beliefs to break free from the self-sabotage cycle.

Principle #14: Ground Your Identity in Christ

Your Identity in Christ

At the outset of this book, I shared my personal story with you about my self-perception. It's a story that has woven its way through my calling as a personal trainer, coach, and someone deeply committed to inspiring others on their path to health and wellness. It's a story of perpetual self-examination, one that led me to gaze into the mirror not with pride in my achievements, gratitude for my health or awe in God's creation of me, but with a critical eye focused mostly on my perceived flaws. For most of my adult life I've dedicated myself daily to workouts, sculpting my muscles and diligently monitoring progress, embracing countless opportunities to boost my health and fitness.

Yet despite the tangible victories there remained an ever-present, relentless self-critique that overshadowed my accomplishments. The mirror was no longer a reflection of the strong and accomplished woman and daughter of God; instead, it magnified cellulite and amplified perceived weaknesses. This pattern extended far beyond the mirror, infiltrating all aspects of my life. Even in the midst of prayer and spiritual devotion, I struggled to see myself as God saw me. When moments of celebration should have been in order, I found myself focusing on areas where I believed I fell short. It seemed as if, despite my strengths, gifts and talents, I had become my harshest judge. Self-acceptance was clouded in self-criticism, obscuring the fullness of who I am. I share this with you because I know I'm not alone in this struggle. I understand that you may have faced a similar inner battle, a conflict between who God says you are and perceived imperfections. Perhaps you're facing it at this moment. We often become our harshest critics, fixating on our own cellulite, both physical and metaphorical, and downplaying the incredible feats we've achieved and the magnificence of our creation.

As we unpack this final principle together, recognize that while this book focuses on releasing physical weight, if it has not already been made clear, the true transformation goes far beyond releasing excess physical weight. It's about unburdening yourself from the emotional weight, characterized by feelings of unworthiness and self-condemnation, that can obscure your true identity in Christ. It's about releasing the mental weight that fuels your constant worry about your weight itself and negative thought patterns that distracts you from God's purpose and peace. These burdens keep you on a hamster wheel, always looking for satisfaction in the wrong places.

Indeed, you will release weight as you apply these principles in this book. However, my heartfelt prayer is that you'll fully embrace this final principle with all your heart and soul: ground your identity in Christ. Without discovering your genuine worth in Him, you may find yourself journeying along a path, only to reach its end and realize you've been on the wrong course. As an avid hiker I know the feeling of putting in the work, the time and the effort, only to have backtrack to the starting point. It's infuriating to say the least.

My hope is to shield you from that experience and guide you toward the liberating understanding that in Christ your identity is unshakable, regardless of your current size. Did you catch that? *Regardless of your size.* God loves you just as you are. Without accepting this truth you'll remain like the Israelites, circling around the same mountain but never entering into the promised land. My hope is that you will come to the truth that you are loved lavishly by God just the way you are right now. There is nothing broken, nothing missing, and nothing lacking in you. When I learned that for myself, it was like a floodgate of freedom opened up.

If you're anything like me, and I think you are if you're still reading, what you're really pursuing is a feeling. The feeling you wrote about in your vision in principle 1: Create Clarity. A feeling of freedom, peace, and joy. Days filled with great meaning, experiences, and memories. In our minds, we believe that if only we looked a certain way, then we would feel X. You can fill in the blank—accomplished, beautiful, successful, happy, worthy, seen, valued, complete. But dear reader, no number on the scale or reflection looking back at you in the mirror will ever bring you satisfaction if your perception of yourself is ground in anything less than who you are in Christ.

> *"We seemed like grasshoppers in our own eyes, and we looked the same to them."* (Numbers 13:33 NIV)

Let's circle back to the negative report of the ten spies in the Book of Numbers. Moses sent twelve spies, one from each tribe, to scout the land of Canaan. Upon their return, there were two conflicting reports.

Joshua and Caleb, representing one group, brought back an optimistic and faith-filled account of the land. They described it as a bountiful and fruitful land that God had promised to give them. Their focus was on the possibility, the promise, and the power of God. In stark contrast, the ten spies painted a picture of fear and hopelessness. They focused on the giants, the fortified cities, and the perceived obstacles. Their report was tainted with fear, doubt, and self-limiting beliefs. The question is, why did they see it this way? Why were these two reports so diametrically opposed to each other?

The spies looked at themselves from a myopic viewpoint and did not see themselves as God saw them. Instead, they viewed themselves as small and insignificant, much like grasshoppers in comparison to the challenges they faced. They were already defeated even before they set out on the exploratory journey because their identity had shaped their reality. Their entire journey through the wilderness showed their fixation on their fears and frustrations instead of fixing their eyes on God. These were the same people who complained at every opportunity and heaved long-suffering sighs at each trifle they endured as Moses led them out of Egypt.

But Joshua and Caleb grounded their identity, and therefore their ability, in God. They didn't deny that the giants were large and the cities near impregnable, but they focused on the God who had vanquished the Egyptians, drowning them in the sea. With God on their side Israel could take the land, they insisted. With God on their side, nothing was impossible.

You, like the twelve spies, also are faced with this choice and opportunity.

You have the power to shape your perception. Will you see yourself as God sees you or will you see yourself as a grasshopper? Will you listen to the voices of the majority who will always be against moving forward to pursue the promises of God or will you move forward in faith, in spite of your fears. I know you will make the right choice. Ground your identity and self-perception in God.

You cannot surpass, out-pace, out-pray, out-exert, or out-diet your self-perception. Sooner or later, a distorted self-image will inevitably guide you back to your initial starting point. That's why God in His infinite wisdom created us in His image so that we can ground our identity in Him. As you understand that you are a beloved child of God, fearfully and wonderfully made, you can start to see yourself as He sees you. You are not defined by your fears, flaws, or past experiences. You are defined by His love and the potential He has placed within you.

The Impact of Limiting Beliefs on Your Identity

Remember the limiting beliefs we discussed in the previous section? We defined them as engrained thoughts, thinking patterns, or beliefs that we hold about ourselves and our world. We recognized that as limiting beliefs become deeply ingrained in our minds and hearts, they act as the silent architects of our self-sabotaging behaviors and emotional struggles.

In this chapter, let's explore the impact of our limiting beliefs and how they can shape our identity if we're not paying attention. When you believe what you believe for long enough, it shapes your reality. It becomes the lens through which you see, believe, and interpret the world around you. It's like walking around with blue sunglasses. The result is that you will constantly see the entire world with a blue haze. We'll call this blue haze or distorted reality your false identity.

Remember the faulty smoke detector? Let's revisit it one final time. If our core fears represent the triggering mechanism that sets off the smoke detector and our limiting beliefs symbolize the malfunctioning wiring, then our false identity is the perceived 'smoke' that is clouding our judgment, perspective, and outlook on everything we do. It's like wearing tinted glasses every day, which affects how we perceive ourselves and the world around us, including our ability to succeed.

Much like smoke and tinted glasses obscure the clarity of our vision, false identities can cloud our understanding of who we truly are. They may make us see ourselves as lesser, unworthy or fundamentally flawed, which can significantly impact our self-esteem and confidence. Just as you would want to clear the smoke to see clearly, addressing and reshaping these false identities is essential to rediscovering your authentic self, grounded in your identity in Christ.

When you live in alignment with God's best for you, your identity begins to transform as you continue to conform to His image and likeness (2 Cor. 3:18). This is a journey of self-discovery and growing in faith. On the other hand, when you live from your false identity—that is, believing lies that don't line up with the Word of God—you inadvertently place constraints on who God designed you to be.

This contrast reminds me of a fable that I came across in my readings.

In the same field stand both a mighty oak tree and a willow tree. The willow tree envies the power and strength that the oak tree possesses. One day a storm, with whipping winds and torrential rain, makes its way through the field. After the storm passes, the willow tree notices that the oak tree has fallen over in the storm. In a state of confusion, she asks the farmer what happened to the oak tree. The farmer tells the willow tree that although the oak was mighty and solid, it was also rigid and inflexible and when the winds were too much for it to resist, the oak tree collapsed under the pressure. The willow thought about herself for a minute. She realized that her ability to survive the storm was due to her flexibility and adaptability, as she was able to bend with the wind to weather the storm. - Author Unknown

What a powerful metaphor for life. Just as the willow tree found strength in its flexibility, you can also discover resilience and stability when you stay connected to Jesus and ground your identity in Him. Christ's teachings, His love, and His grace provide us with the spiritual foundation that allows us to bend, adapt, and endure the storms of life with unwavering faith. By anchoring your identity in Him, you find the strength to withstand the challenges that come your way and emerge from adversity even stronger, just like the willow tree standing tall after the storm has passed.

Alignment

When you're not in alignment with who God calls you to be, you can inadvertently find yourself aligning with other influences—your past, the enemy's whispers, or societal expectations—and this can have a detrimental impact on your health and your weight.

I can look back and see how all three of these impacted me at various points in my life and informed many of my decisions. As a survivor of sexual abuse at a young age, I developed very mixed feelings about my body. It was something to be desired by others, yet it was something that I did not have any power over. These mixed messages led me to adopt many extremes and self-indulgences while growing up. This internal struggle not only affected my self-image but also influenced my relationship with food and my overall approach to health.

This experience also opened the door to allow the enemy to continue to remind me of my brokenness and powerlessness. Unwittingly, I believed his lies for many years. I lived with my secret shame and often found temporary comfort in unhealthy distractions such as food and television. As I sought counseling, I learned that I am not defined by my past and I am not the person the enemy whispers about in my head. I am not who society says I am. Yes, I may have roles as a personal trainer, a health coach, a mother, wife, and sister, but at the end of the day I am a child of God. Period! I am not lacking, I am not missing anything, and I am not broken.

By the end of this chapter my hope is that you, too, will embrace this truth for yourself.

For now, I want to paint a clear picture of how these false identities may have found their way into your life.

Let's look at how these three influences may have impacted your life and your health journey:

Your Past:

During our formative years, when we are impressionable and unable to distinguish truth from falsehood, events or messages can deeply impact the way we perceive ourselves and the world around us. These influential moments can give rise to what we call limiting or faulty beliefs.

At this tender stage of life, everything we see and hear is absorbed into our fragile subconscious minds, where it is imprinted as absolute truth. As we mature these limiting beliefs persist in the background, often triggering unconscious reactions and behaviors. Over time they can forge false identities, leading us down paths that deviate from the person God intended us to be.

These beliefs are like heavy baggage we carry from our past. Past experiences, traumas, and negative self-perceptions can deeply mold our sense of self and our behaviors. The weight of previous failures, emotional wounds, or unhealthy habits can cast a long shadow over our present choices. For example, unresolved issues from our past may manifest as emotional eating or self-sabotage in our attempts to achieve better health and a healthier weight.

When we fail to align our lives with God's vision for our well-being, these burdens from our past can negatively affect our health. In essence, it's a continuous cycle—the limiting beliefs formed in our impressionable years and the baggage of our past experiences intertwine to shape our identity and influence our present choices, including those related to our health and weight.

The Enemy's Influence:

The enemy, Satan, employs every conceivable tactic, utilizing even our unique personalities and God-given gifts to ensnare us. He seeks to taint and corrupt every good thing bestowed upon us by God. His most potent weapon is psychological deception, a sinister scheme designed to convince us of our inferiority, inadequacy and worthlessness, especially in the eyes of God.

When we are not watchful and vigilant, the enemy plants insidious doubts, fears, and temptations into our minds. These influences can gradually steer us away from God's intended path, leading us astray. They may manifest as unhealthy cravings, reminders of your past failures and weaknesses, self-destructive behaviors, or a lack of self-worth. Succumbing to these harmful influences takes a toll on both our physical and emotional well-being.

Lastly, Societal Expectations:

Society often bombards us with unrealistic beauty standards, promotes a pervasive diet culture, and extols superficial ideals of success. These societal pressures can be relentless, and when we succumb to them instead of aligning with our true identity in Christ we may find ourselves ensnared in a cycle of extreme diets, body-shaming, and other harmful practices as we strive to meet these unattainable standards.

This struggle is real! The allure of the world can be strong, and if we're not careful it can dictate the kind of person we should be. It will also lead you to crash diets and extreme weight loss measures. When we veer away from alignment with who God has called us to be, we often end up conforming to the molds shaped by the world. In the absence of our spiritual compass guiding us to our Heavenly Father, we inadvertently reflect a diminished version of ourselves.

As we journey through this final chapter together, we'll explore the connection between your spiritual alignment and your health. When you root your identity in God's love and purpose for you, you gain the strength and wisdom to make healthier choices. You can find the grace to forgive yourself for past mistakes and let go of self-destructive patterns. You can resist the negative influences of the enemy and society, focusing instead on your well-being as a cherished child of God.

Identity Theft

In this day and age, identity theft is a real problem. Although I've never experienced it myself, I know someone who did and they suffered not only from the economic impact, but the emotional and psychological impact lasted for a long time after the original incident.

Identity theft is a fairly new problem in our age of technology, but it has been going on for thousands of years and it started in the Garden of Eden. Satan used the serpent to trick Adam and Eve into doubting their true identity as children of the Most High God. He planted seeds of doubt in their minds so they would doubt God's love for them. He made them question their rights and privileges as children of God and their dominion to rule over the Earth with unlimited access to God (Genesis 1:26).

Since then, Satan continues to try to deceive us by having us not see our true identity. The Bible is replete with characters who struggled with identity. Satan even tried to use the same tactics on Jesus Himself (Matthew 4:3 –10). This is what we've been building up to up until this point. This was always Satan's goal. He will always attack our identity in Christ. When he can get us to question who we are and whose we are, he's won. And this is where you find yourself right now.

But God's Word is clear on your identity.

It says, "*So God created man in his own image, in the image of God he created him; male and female he created them*" (Genesis 1:27).

Thankfully, through faith in the life, death, and resurrection of Jesus, we can ground our identity in our Lord and Savior. We have been transformed from a rebellious people into reflections of our Savior.

Jesus said in John 10:10: "*The thief comes only in order to steal and kill and destroy. I came that they may have and enjoy life, and have it in abundance.*" (AMPC)

Isaiah 43:1 says, "*Fear not, for I have redeemed you; I have called you by name, you are mine*" (RSV). You are saved from living out of a false identity. You don't have to identify with your sin nature but rather with the bloodline of Jesus Christ.

Let's look at how one of God's anointed struggled and overcame the stronghold of false identity and achieved his breakthrough.

> "*But now, this is what the LORD says— he who created you, Jacob, he who formed you, Israel: "Do not fear, for I have redeemed you; I have summoned you by name; you are mine."*" (Isaiah 43:1 NIV)

Let's look again in the Bible to understand how your past and your limiting beliefs give way to the unhealthy creation of false identities.

Nowhere in the Bible is there a better example of living out of your false identity than in the story of Jacob.

Jacob's struggles began in the womb! His parents, Isaac and Rebekah, named him "Jacob" which means "supplanter or deceiver" in Hebrew. The word "supplant" means "to overthrow by tripping up—to supersede by treachery."

Why would they name him this? The Bible says that Jacob wrestled with his older twin brother while he was in his mother Rebekah's womb. (Gen 25:21-27) At the time of his birth, he grasped the heel of older brother as if he were trying to take his brother's place as first-born. You see a glimpse of what could have been a powerful, natural gift—Jacob was a fighter. But you'll also see how the improper nurturing of this gift led to many difficulties down the road for him. I wonder what difference it would have made in his life if his parents named him something different!

You may also have been born with the cards stacked against you. You may have been born in a single parent household, in poverty, in chaos all around you. Maybe both of your parents were overweight or had a host of pre-existing health conditions. If that's your story, know that, like Jacob, despite what you were born, God has a divine purpose and promise for you (Genesis 35: 10-11). Jacob's story, like your own, will be a tale of transformation and victory.

The first thirty-plus years of Jacob's life were spent living out of his false identity as a supplanter. In Genesis 25:27-34, after grabbing his brother's heel at birth, the second recorded action of Jacob is when he manipulates his brother into giving his birthright over to him. We continue to see Jacob's downward spiral in chapter 27, this time encouraged by his mother Rebekah. In this next act of deception, Jacob deceives his father Isaac by disguising himself as his older brother, thereby stealing his twin brother's blessing (an honor that a father bestows upon his eldest son before passing on).

Fast forward the story and Jacob then leaves in fear of his older brother, only to get caught up in more deception. He agrees to work for seven years for his uncle in exchange for his uncle's daughter Rachel's hand in marriage. True to his identity, he is now deceived by his uncle who tricks him into working an additional seven years after switching brides on his wedding night!

Despite all his brokenness and deception, God is always with Jacob because of the covenant he made with his forefathers Abraham and Issac. As tensions continue to mount while he lives with his uncle, two wives and all that he has amassed, God speaks to Jacob and tells him to return home and promises him that He will be with him (Genesis 31:3).

In spite of his fears, Jacob obeys God and packs up his family and sets off to return home to face his brother who he betrayed.

A strange but powerful event takes place on his way home. While traveling, for an unspoken reason, he decides to stay alone in the dark of the night. During this night, the Bible says a stranger finds Jacob and begins to wrestle with him all night long. This is no ordinary man because with a single touch the stranger (an angel of the Lord) dislocated Jacob's hip. Isn't it amazing how God met Him at the place of his true identity—a wrestler!

> *"So Jacob was left alone, and a man wrestled with him till daybreak. When the man saw that he could not overpower him, he touched the socket of Jacob's hip so that his hip was wrenched as he wrestled with the man. Then the man said, "Let me go, for it is daybreak."*
>
> *But Jacob replied, "I will not let you go unless you bless me."*
>
> *The man asked him, "What is your name?"*
>
> *Then the man said, "Your name will no longer be Jacob, but Israel, because you have struggled with God and with humans and have overcome." Genesis 32:24-28 (NIV)*

It is God who gives Jacob a new name and a new identity. He is transformed from Jacob which means supplanter or deceiver, to Israel—one who wrestles with God and is victorious. This is a return to his true identity.

You might be feeling like Jacob. You know that God has a plan for your life. You have spent so much of your life living out of your false identity, trying to figure things out the best way you know how. Like Jacob, you realize that you're trying to figure things out in your own strength.

This is why you're here right now. You have been wrestling with God, you have struggled in your false identity, and you're ready to move past the shame and the guilt of your past and let God give you a new name. You're ready to stand on His promises and believe that you are who God says you are.

Like Jacob, it's time to acknowledge your true identity, gifts, and passions. You'll also understand how your unchecked fears and limiting beliefs have caused your gifts to go amiss.

Addressing False Identities in Your Health Journey: The 3-Step Reset

By now, I hope you have gained a better understanding of how false identities can hinder you from perceiving yourself as God sees you and how it's been impacting your weight-releasing journey.

As we get close to the end of this transformative journey, let's revisit our 3-Step Reset together one final time so you can learn how to reframe your false identities.

Step 1: Pause

Whereas all the other pauses through this book were helpful to allow you to pay attention and change your mental state in moments of anxiety or misalignment, this final pause will be guided and structured. It will require you to carve out some time to sit quietly and pay attention to how you feel about yourself and your ability to succeed.

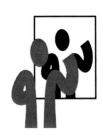

You will need a journal for your thoughts.

Sit quietly and return to your box breathing. Inhale: Close your eyes and take a slow, deep breath in through your nose for a count of 5. Feel the air filling your lungs and expanding your chest. Hold: Hold your breath for another count of 5. This is a moment of stillness where you can center your thoughts and focus inward. Exhale: Slowly exhale through your mouth for a count of 5, releasing any tension or stress. Pause: After exhaling, pause for a final count of 5. During this moment, simply be present and acknowledge the presence of God. Repeat 4-5 times

Step 2: Pray

Incorporate this prayer into your daily routine. Select a specific time that works best for you, either upon waking in the morning or before you go to bed each night. Consistency is key to making it a habit.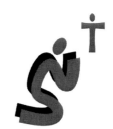

Read the prayer slowly and reflect on each statement. Allow the words to resonate with your heart and spirit.

You can personalize the prayer by adding specific details, concerns, or expressions of gratitude as you feel led.

Commit to praying this prayer daily to reinforce the affirmations and foster a deep connection with God.

Consider keeping a journal to jot down any insights, feelings, or experiences that arise during or after your prayer time.

Heavenly Father,

I come before You with a heart full of gratitude for Your boundless love and acceptance. I believe that I am unconditionally loved by You, regardless of my flaws and past mistakes. Your love is the unshakable foundation of my identity, a love that transcends my imperfections and reminds me that I am cherished beyond measure.

I trust in Your purpose and plan for my life, knowing that Your guidance is unwavering and Your direction is sure. As I navigate my journey, I find confidence in Your divine purpose, which provides clarity amidst life's uncertainties.

I release the burden of guilt and self-condemnation, for I can forgive myself for my past failures and mistakes. Your grace is more than sufficient, offering me the space for forgiveness and renewal.

I recognize that I am fearfully and wonderfully made, a masterpiece intricately designed by Your loving hands. My uniqueness is not a flaw but a testament to Your intentional craftsmanship.

With humility, I am aware of my strengths and gifts, and I commit to using them to serve You and others. These talents are tools to bring glory to Your name and to bless those around me.

I resist the trap of comparison, understanding that You have carved a unique path for my life. I trust in the significance of my journey, for it is purposefully designed by Your hand.

I believe in the constancy and unwavering nature of Your love, regardless of my circumstances. In every season of life Your love remains my steadfast anchor, sustaining me through it all.

I choose to treat myself with kindness and compassion, recognizing that I am valued by You. The grace and compassion You shower upon me I extend to myself, acknowledging my intrinsic value as Your beloved child.

As a vessel of Your love and grace, I embrace my role in impacting the lives of others positively. May my actions and words reflect Your love, bringing light and hope to those I encounter.

I find my identity firmly rooted in Christ, unshaken by the opinions of others. It is in Him that I discover my true self, transcending the fleeting judgments of the world.

In grounding my identity in You, I experience a deep sense of peace and contentment. I rest in the assurance that I am beloved, secure, and deeply loved by You.

Thank You for this transformative journey, and I pray that I may continue to grow in Your truth and grace. In Jesus' Name, I pray. Amen.

Step 3: Practice

For this final Active Practice, I suggest you place your hand over your heart as you receive this prayer.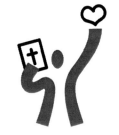

I pray that this concluding chapter has served as a mirror, reflecting the growth and transformation you've experienced throughout this journey. As you read this prayer daily, may it resonate within your heart, guiding you to ground your identity in Christ and affirming your worth as His beloved child. Your identity is unshakable, firmly rooted in the unwavering love and grace of our Heavenly Father. Your victory is at hand!

Principle 14 Summary

Reflect on these key points:

- Your identity can be shaped by long-held limiting beliefs, creating a false self-image. These false identities are like tinted glasses, clouding your perspective and self-perception, often leading to a negative self-image.

- To overcome false identities, you must ground your identity in Christ and align with God's vision for your well-being.

- The 3-Step Reset—Pause, Pray, and Active Practice—can help address false identities.

The Secret to Weight Loss Breakthroughs, God's Way

In the midst of Ontario's harsh winters, where the landscape often appears as though it has been through a battle, with fallen trees obstructing the path, it's remarkable to witness the resilience of nature. Despite the challenges, new hope emerges every spring as life bursts forth in a triumphant display of vitality and renewal.

Just like the tenacity of the trees on the Bruce Trail, you too have faced your personal struggles and obstacles on your journey to better health and weight release. You've encountered setbacks, roadblocks, and moments when it felt like the odds were against you. Just as nature perseveres and flourishes, however, so can you. Embrace the changing seasons of your life, knowing that with every spring a new beginning awaits. Your own journey to health and well-being is a testament to the power of resilience, determination, and the unwavering faith that you can, and will, thrive. Your story is a testament to the beauty of transformation, and it's a living testament to the fact that, with God's guidance, you will achieve your healthy weight. God's way.

Always remember that your health journey is symbolic of your personal journey back to Him. It's your adventure through the thickets and forests of your life, learning how to blaze the trail set before you. It's about releasing the burdens that have weighed you down—emotionally, spiritually, and physically. You may have sought answers in diets, exercise regimens, and countless strategies, but the true answer lies in returning to God and aligning your journey with His way. He invites you to lay down your burdens, including those related to weight and health, and find rest in His grace and guidance.

You've created your vision for where you want to go and you've got your blueprint for how you're going to get there, so now it's time to start blazing your trail. You've got everything you need, and I promise you that you will never need another weight loss book if you choose to listen to the Father's gentle voice. A voice that lovingly guides your steps.

You now know the secret to your breakthrough. It's your journey back to God. As you take each step, keep reminding yourself that it's not just about reaching a destination but a continual drawing to Abba Father as He draws near to you. In His presence, you find the answers not only to weight loss but to everything that weighs you down in life.

May you continue to move towards your vision as you prioritize maximizing your energy and stewarding your temple. In doing so you will walk in His light, reflecting His glory. And the added bonus is that your body will naturally find its right size.

Keep on learning and growing, but remember to do it all from a place of rest. I've been guilty of reading a book and hastily moving on to the next one, failing to fully grasp the precious insights the Lord intended for me. Let's adopt a posture of what I refer to as "relaxed intensity". The weight of expectations, pressures, and the endless pursuit of perfection can be heavy burdens to bear. In Matthew 11:28, Jesus invites us to come to Him, all who are weary and burdened, and He promises to give us rest. Embrace this rest as you continue your journey to health, knowing that it's not about the destination but the transformative path you're on. As you walk in the assurance of God's love and grace, with a heart at rest, you'll discover that your health journey is not a burden but a beautiful adventure filled with growth, discovery, and the joyful anticipation of what lies ahead.

I still have a very long way to go to complete my hike along the Bruce Trail. Much like my Bruce Trail you have a path that has been laid out for you, and your assignment is to follow it. Know that it will be a journey filled with moments of growth, self-discovery, and transformation. Embrace each step, each challenge, and each success as a part of your adventure. Keep your eyes on the destination, but don't forget to savor the beauty of the trail. With determination and faith you'll continue your progress, and may your path be blessed with strength, resilience, and the peace that comes from walking it with Him by your side.

The Journey Continues...

As we journeyed through the pages of this book together, I pray that you discovered the remarkable transformations that aligning your faith with your health can bring into your life. But our exploration doesn't end here. In this special supplemental section, you have the privilege of meeting eleven extraordinary coaches, each with their own stories of triumph and trials, struggles, and successes. They have walked the path of faith and health, and their unique insights will help make your path even clearer, inspiring you to keep moving toward your goals.

These phenomenal women have gone on to become leading coaches and experts in their field, driven by a commitment to pay it forward. Coaches are the unsung champions of growth and development. They don't just hoard the lessons they've learned for themselves; they're driven by a deep desire to share their knowledge and experiences with others. These humble servants stand in the gap, extending a helping hand to guide and support those on their own journeys.

Coaches are marked by their transparency and their genuine heart to serve, making them invaluable allies in your health journey. In this bonus chapter, you'll have the privilege of getting to know eleven such extraordinary coaches who have been trained in the Breakthrough Method and are blazing new trails. Their stories are testaments to the power of faith, health, and community in achieving remarkable personal growth and freedom. They have embraced the role of coach as a calling, and their dedication to helping others is nothing short of inspiring. Be encouraged.

My Journey of Inner Transformation

Coach Jaime M. Speligene

Alone in the house, I stood in my bathroom, staring blankly into the mirror. My expression was a mix of emptiness and disorientation. The reality cut deep as I tried to decipher the image gazing back at me. I simply turned and walked away, disgusted at the unrecognizable person I had become. How did this happen? How had I evolved into this frumpy, pale, wrinkled, exhausted, overweight, shell of a woman I once knew? Where had I gone? I had become a battered and shattered version of myself, lost in the aftermath of life's hardships and my coping methods. Despite medication, depression had become my constant companion, and food my primary source of comfort. Every aspect of my life was out of alignment and out of control. I finally hit rock bottom!

"Enough!" I screamed as loud as I could— a desperate plea crying out to the Lord as I continued praying, pleading, and begging for guidance or hope. Tears welled up, streaming down my face and filling my palms as I let my entire body fall to the ground, collapsing helplessly into a child's pose. I was hysterical and it wouldn't stop anytime soon. I couldn't endure this anymore! I was completely desperate for recovery and restoration. I cried out for the resurgence of my faith, health, and purpose. I needed renewal and transformation inside and out. This was NOT going to be my story.

Back in 2015 we faced the overwhelming decision to uproot our family, leaving behind the familiar and those we held dearest for my husband's career. Coming off three months of total bedrest for my now-six-week-old son, I stood there sobbing while embracing those who had loved, supported, and helped us the most. Accompanied by my husband, a ten-year-old, a two-year-old, and an infant, we began a journey spanning 800 miles, venturing into the unfamiliar. Prayerfully we chose this path, one that would challenge our resilience and strength in dealing with change and distance.

Now settled in a new town and state, I knew no one. I even had to use the GPS on my phone to find the grocery store only a few miles from the house. Additionally, there was the loneliness that came with having a husband constantly traveling with his new position. It all weighed heavily on me. His frequent absence left a void in our home, and certainly in my life. In the quiet moments of the evenings insecurities crept in, slowly draining my confidence. I found myself crippled by my own thoughts, conjuring up hypothetical scenarios that only made me question my relationship and worth. The isolation created an easy opportunity for emotional binge-eating sessions at night in a desperate attempt to fill the emptiness, silence, and the anxious whispers in my mind. Each bite seemed to momentarily relieve the feelings of lonesomeness, but it was a fleeting source of comfort, followed by hours of guilt and regret which I would then numb with mindless scrolling on my phone or binge-watching TV. It was a chaotic cycle, and the words "self-care" didn't even occur to me.

During those challenging days, life as a mom felt like a game of survival. Relentless lack of sleep kept me in a perpetual haze, clouding my every thought and action. I tried to navigate the demanding role of being a cook, maid, nurse, room mom, chauffeur, educator, shopper, money manager— all while barely able to keep my eyes open. My cravings spiraled out of control, and my go-to became all things quick, processed, leftover, and non-nutritious. Then there was my persistent addiction to Dr. Pepper, a source of quick energy upon which I leaned on far more that I should have. It became my main source of hydration and nutrition starting at around 9 am. While I tirelessly tried to nurse and nourish my newborn, I neglected to nourish myself. My own body's needs were completely taking a backseat to the demands of what felt like single motherhood. The struggle to find balance amid this emotional whirlwind was a steep uphill battle that I didn't have the resources, courage, or energy to climb.

In this season in my life, one pivotal event stands out vividly—The Fall. It was a life-changing moment when sheer fatigue blurred my vision, causing me to miss a step and take a perilous stumble, face first, down a half-flight of wooden stairs with my precious six-month-old in my arms. The thud of the fall was a symphony of fear and shooting pain; I couldn't feel my legs. I was home alone with all three children, and my husband, family, and friends were all hundreds of miles away. Yelling for my oldest child to come and get the unharmed baby, it took what seemed like forever to feel and move my toes and legs. I was in shock, terrified, and knew this would ultimately change everything.

The aftermath was a harsh reality of severe back pain, walking with a cane, and feeling like I was 80 at just 40. It was difficult to get myself and my children in and out of the car. I could barely push a stroller. I couldn't play with my kids or do most normal physical activities a healthy mom would do. It took all I had to accomplish the basic needs of my home and family. The injury demanded rigorous physical therapy, traction therapy, and multiple cortisone injections in my spine. It was a grueling process extending over a year to regain my mobility and strength. From this setback, I mustered the determination to stage a comeback, refusing to let this define my future. It was a wake-up call and has become my testament to the human spirit's capacity to rise, even from the most challenging of falls… literally.

During my physical recovery, I discovered a devotional that instantly resonated with me on the Holy Bible app: *Weight Loss, God's Way*. The words immediately struck a chord within me from that very first devotion. I sensed from the very beginning that this was different—something that had the potential to reshape me from the inside out. On day 2 of the devotional, October 13, 2021, the exercise was to write "My Why" — the reason for sticking to this process and my goals. I wrote:

> *"The cost is my quality of life in everything I do. I don't want my children to struggle with their health or weight, and I don't want to be the example of 'do as I say, not as I do'. I will never be physically healed, and I will always live in fear of my next diagnosis. I will never experience full freedom, joy, or peace of mind. I will continue to look and feel disgusting. I will continue to be embarrassed around people and insecure that my husband will leave or cheat. NOTHING GOOD COMES FROM STAYING THE SAME!"*

I read this every morning for motivation to keep going. It helped me stick to the program and to the work. I began embarking on prayer walks—a tangible sign of my physical progress. I found strength in weak emotional moments by creating recorded "Scripture Pep-Talks" with empowering Bible verses and prayers that I could easily access at any time. I would place my hand over my heart and pray before I was about to engage in destructive eating behavior. Slowly but surely, I was changing.

Weight Loss, God's Way became a compass, guiding me towards discovering God's vision for my life through seeking His will and alignment with the Holy Spirit in a way I'd never fully experienced before. It propelled me to redefine myself, time, and resources by establishing clear priorities and values. I actively practiced and immersed myself in the daily devotions, worksheets, accountability, and regular check-ins. I began to realize the significance of nurturing my relationship with God and myself, enabling me to be the best mother and wife I could be. I embraced the method wholeheartedly, understanding that perfection was not the goal, but rather persistence. *Weight Loss, God's Way* became my path toward a brighter, purpose-filled life. It took over a year, but it was undeniably one of the healthiest and best years of my life.

The culmination of this transformative journey was the Breakthrough Celebration—an awe-inspiring experience where I met remarkable women from the *Weight Loss, God's Way* community who inspired and uplifted me. Taking the stage and being recognized for my initial 35-pound weight release was a moment of immense pride and a validation of my achievements. I was closer to God, mentally healthier, and physically stronger than I had been in almost a decade. I cherish the ongoing relationships and support this community has brought into my life. The element of faith has made all the difference in my transformation, serving as a steadfast anchor through life's continual trials and tribulations. Its principles gave me hope and strength, enabling me to navigate challenges with resilience and determination. Having come this far, I now stand ready to extend my hand to others on their journey. I'm eager to share my experiences, offer support, and light the path for those seeking their own transformation, fueled by faith, perseverance, and the unwavering belief that change is possible. As a coach trained in the Breakthrough Method, my commitment to my clients is unwavering, and my passion to guide them towards their full potential knows no bounds. I have witnessed the powerful changes that are within their reach, and I look forward to helping them others get there.

My Journey to Rebuilding My Temple, God's Way

Coach Stephanie L. Franklin-Suber

God is a divine tripartite being—Father, Son, and Holy Spirit. Just as His Temple in Jerusalem reflected His tripartite being (outer court, inner court, and innermost court), we, as His human temples, are tripartite beings (body, soul, and spirit).

Destruction of My Temple (Body, Soul, and Spirit).

My Body Destroyed by Medical Trauma

In 2006, at the age of 48, I was diagnosed with a rare form of breast cancer. The doctors offered a grim prognosis, giving me a maximum of five years to live. Cancer had claimed my mother at the age of 49, and it seemed that history was set to repeat itself.

As we walked through the valley of the shadow of death, my husband and I turned to God to lead us. I immersed myself in the healing scriptures and fervently prayed to Jehovah Rapha, my Healer, for my physical healing. My deepest desire was to witness our son graduate from college. God answered our prayers. Grateful for my husband's unwavering love and support, against all medical odds I stand here today by God's grace, alive and cancer-free.

Yet the journey was far from over. Surgery, chemotherapy, radiation, and an array of other intensive treatments and medications took a heavy toll on my body. Despite my survival, my body was ravaged by long term side effects.

Undeterred, I attempted to resume my high-stress career as an attorney in 2007. I struggled, for my body had undergone dramatic change due to medical trauma. The more I pushed, the more the stress impeded my recovery. God was signaling that I had to relinquish my career, but it was intertwined with my identity. My body was saying "no". I, however, refused to listen.

In 2012, the ground crumbled beneath my feet.

My Soul Destroyed by Emotional Trauma

My youngest sister's sudden death from a cardiac arrhythmia, coupled with her husband's suicide a month later, shook my soul. They were both in their forties. In my grief and sorrow, guilt gnawed at me. I felt that I had missed the signs of my sister's emotional eating and my brother-in-law's contemplation of suicide.

The medical and emotional traumas manifested in my body, giving rise to an onslaught of chronic illnesses and conditions that persist to this day.

By 2013, heart and pulmonary complications forced me into medical disability. I was incessantly battling chronic infection, inflammation, and lymphedema. My immune system and microbiome faltered. The limbic system in my brain was impaired, leading to chemical intolerance, multiple chemical sensitivities, and hypersensitivity to environmental changes.

It took six long years to stabilize my physical health. Ongoing health challenges compelled me to shift my priorities from my career to my health. I had to adapt to numerous lifestyle and environmental limitations which kept me home bound.

As I was beginning to find stability, the pandemic struck in 2019.

My Spirit Destroyed by Emotional Eating

During the pandemic lockdown, my life and my weight spiraled out of control.

Emotional eating and "yo-yo" weight fluctuations had plagued me for years, but I lacked clarity and awareness on the root causes and triggers.

I had experimented with countless diets, pills, supplements, and exercise regimens, veering between starvation and bingeing. However, during the pandemic lockdown, the emotional eating escalated to an alarming new level. Fear, panic, and uncertainty consumed me. We were isolated from family and community, unable to visit loved ones in nursing homes or gather for funerals.

I lost perspective, magnifying the circumstances instead of magnifying God, His power, and His unfailing love. I plummeted into a deep pit of paralyzing fear, despair, and depression.

In a matter of a few months, I gained 50 pounds. My weight ballooned to the heaviest I had ever been. I had breathing problems, joint pain, and trouble navigating stairs and doing simple tasks. I slept poorly and barely moved. I tried to escape the pain by watching TV, online shopping, and self-soothing through food. I stuffed my feelings in secret and mastered "contact-less" take-out and delivery, ordering almost every day. My shame grew as restaurant staff and delivery drivers began recognizing me by name.

The more I ate and the more weight I gained, the deeper I sank into the darkness of shame, guilt, and self-loathing. Toxic thoughts and emotions engulfed me, leaving me feeling hopeless and helpless.

The pandemic lockdown gave me an excuse to hide from family and friends. I also hid from God. While I knew Him as Jehovah Rapha, my Healer, who had cured my body of cancer, I believed that my weight was solely within my control. I just needed more willpower and self-control!

Then God stepped in and rescued me from the pit.

Rebuilding My Temple from the Inside Out Through the Breakthrough Method

In December 2020, as I desperately searched for hope, God led me to *Weight Loss, God's Way (WLGW)*. Yet again, I was on a quest for the perfect weight loss book or self-help tool to fix me. It was no coincidence that I discovered

Cathy Morenzie's book, *Weight Loss, God's Way* and the online program and membership community at weightlossgodsway.com.

I embarked on the "21-Day Challenge," and, taking a leap of faith, joined the program in January 2021, and then took the transformative "Breakthrough" course.

My Spirit Restored by Cultivating My Relationship with God

The cornerstone of my transformation was the "Reveal the Root–Clarity" principle, which uncovered unmet emotional needs that I had long ignored and avoided. Instead of processing painful emotions and turning to God for comfort, I had suppressed medical and emotional traumas. I had denied grief, loss, and guilt.

My weight loss goal was to shed 50 pounds, and for ten months I made steady progress. I adhered to my healthy boundaries of intermittent fasting, meal planning, food tracking, and daily exercise. In October 2021, I proudly reached my goal weight. However, I relapsed a month later and regained fifteen pounds over the holidays. I was disappointed and discouraged, but I knew that God had led me to WLGW. Quitting was not an option.

I resumed my journey in January 2022, this time with a different perspective. The relapse caused me to self-examine and gain clarity. I had reverted to old habits of perfectionism and control, fixating on the numbers on the scale, the measurements, the tools, and the progress checkmarks. I had lost sight of keeping God at the forefront of my journey.

Instead of hiding from God, I began cultivating my relationship with Him through daily devotions, prayer, meditation, and Bible study. I learned to surrender and acknowledge that He was in control of EVERYTHING. I admitted that I desperately needed His guidance and strength every step of the way.

While I acknowledged my progress, I realized that God's work in me was far from finished.

My Soul Restored by Accountability, Coaching, and Community

I enlisted individual WLGW coaching for additional guidance and support.

My coach helped me view the relapse as an opportunity for self-discovery. I was motivated to modify my habits and mindsets. I practiced renewing my mind with God's Word to reinforce positive beliefs and adopt new thought patterns. I embraced the fellowship of the WLGW membership community. My focus expanded from my weight releasing journey to my faith journey with God.

I developed a heightened awareness of the emotional triggers that led to emotional eating and bingeing. I learned to recognize when old, unhealthy habits and coping mechanisms resurface, threatening to take me out of alignment with God's best for me.

My Body Restored by Healthy Eating, Exercise, and Rest

After ups and downs, I triumphantly reached my goal weight once more in May 2022. My weight and body composition remain stable. I follow a consistent and sustainable action plan encompassing healthy eating, regular exercise, stress management, and ample rest.

Reclaiming A Life of Health and Wholeness

Awareness served as the catalyst for my breakthrough. The holistic approach of the *Breakthrough Method*—integrating body, soul, and spirit—was essential to my transformation.

It is imperative to confront core fears, unmet emotional needs, limiting beliefs, false identities, and unhealthy habits. Only God can satisfy those needs and love us into health and wholeness. His divine will is that we experience health and wholeness so that we can serve Him and fulfill His divine plan.

God is the source of our hope. The key is to trust His will, His ways, and His timing, surrendering our journey to Him each day, holding nothing back. Our focus must be on God, not ourselves. The journey is not about our willpower or failures. It is about God and what He desires to do in and through us. He created us and He knows us better than we know ourselves.

The journey entails letting go of the past and allowing God to guide, teach and heal you, trusting His goodness, faithfulness, and power in the process. As God molds and shapes you for greater service to Him, keep moving forward with Him in faith. Moment by moment, step by step, day by day—in alignment with Him in body, soul, and spirit.

In sharing my story, I hope to inspire women facing similar struggles with a message of hope. My journey has led me to become a Christian Health Coach, using my past pain to empower others seeking wholeness in body, soul, and spirit.

I am one of God's miracles, a testament to His healing power and transformative grace.

My Journey from Perfectionism to Grace and Healing

Coach Denise McKerlie

There I am. That's me, the chubby girl in the front row. I can say that about all my school pictures. From first grade through high school, I was teased mercilessly about my weight.

In my family, food was at the center of what we did. My parents were a part of the "clean your plate" club. After all, there were starving children all over the world who would love to have what we had. I grew up next door to one set of grandparents and a mile down the road from the other set. Home-made cookies, candies, cakes, and pies were always available. Special foods were made for birthdays and holidays, so I learned to equate food with love. It was Grandma's love language.

I entered high school at almost 200 pounds and topped the scale at 275 by the time I finished college. Throughout my adulthood, I tried all the diets. Nutrisystem, Weight Watchers, the cabbage soup diet, the Mayo Clinic 3-day diet, vegetarian, vegan, keto, shots, pills...the list goes on and on. I'd do okay for a while, then fall off the program and the weight would come back on.

On top of being labeled "morbidly obese" I was diagnosed with depression, anxiety, high blood pressure, elevated cholesterol and triglycerides, and pre-diabetes. The stress in my life was tremendous and food was my comfort. After losing my husband of 17 years in December of 2016, the depression and anxiety reached a critical point. Although I was no longer his caregiver, my stress level remained high, and I eventually suffered a nervous breakdown.

Food became even more of a solace for me and the number on the scale continued to climb until I reached almost 340 pounds. I turned to the medical field to try to lose weight and, although I had a little success at first, I eventually returned to my old ways. "There has to be a better way," I thought to myself. I just couldn't go on the way I was. I avoided stairs at all costs, rode in a mobility scooter to do my shopping, couldn't walk much at all, and felt like I'd never enjoy life and do all the things I had dreamed of doing.

Then, in January of 2022, I discovered some inspirational, thought-provoking devotions by Cathy Morenzie on the YouVersion Bible app on my phone. They talked about a different approach to weight release, one that included God. I had been a Christian from the age of 10, but had never included God other than to say, "Okay, God, I'm doing this diet. Please help me." I had to find out more.

I enrolled in the *Weight Loss, God's Way* (WLGW) challenges and my life began to change from the inside out. At the end of the challenge, I knew that God had led me to this program and that this was the answer to my constant battle with weight. I signed up for the next WLGW program and hired a WLGW coach. Every day, the thought-provoking lessons spoke to me and inspired me to turn my journey over to God first and allow him to lead me rather than trying to find the next greatest weight-loss thing and drag God along, hoping it would work.

This way was different. I surrendered my depressed, anxious, morbidly obese way of life to God and asked Him to show me the path to take. God showed up in a mighty way and gave me strength each day. Through all the devotions, I learned about how my past hurts, fears, and limiting beliefs were holding me back. I turned these all over to God, and He healed me and showed me who I was in His eyes.

Throughout my life, I said so many things and developed so many beliefs that were keeping me captive: "I'm just supposed to be overweight", "I've always been overweight", "It's in my genetics to be overweight", "I'll never lose all the weight", and the big one: "If you can't do it right the first time, don't do it at all."

Perfectionism. Oh boy, that was me to a "T". It was drilled into me as a child, and my self-worth was wrapped in it. If I did things perfectly, I was worthy; if I made mistakes, I was unworthy. Unworthy of love, praise, or acceptance. Perfectionism became a way of gaining these things because I thought I was not accepted because of my physical appearance. I had to be the best at everything: A's on all my school work, first place in any competition, knowledgeable about everything, house in perfect order. If I couldn't do things perfectly I experienced guilt, which led to more depression and anxiety and more eating.

Through *Weight Loss, God's Way*, God began to heal me of the need to be perfect and show me that my self-worth is determined by who I am through Christ and not what I do. Giving myself grace and accepting myself with all my flaws has been life-changing in all areas of my life, including my weight-release journey. God impressed in my heart that I am "fearfully and wonderfully made" (Psalms 139:14, NIV) in His image.

My life began to change from the inside out as I leaned into God and embraced all that He was teaching me. Healing those past hurts and habits not only led to better emotional health, but also to better physical health. The numbers began to change on the scale. In a year, I not only released 80 pounds but I also released toxic thoughts that had kept me captive. When I ate something outside of my boundaries or missed a day of exercise, I gave myself grace and made better choices the next time. I no longer had the "I'll start again on Monday" mentality. One mistake didn't mean that I had failed, it simply meant that I was human. I turned it over to God and chose to stay the course.

Staying the course brought about so many wins in my life: I can shop all day without getting exhausted, I can shop "off the rack", I can walk a 5K, I am no longer labeled morbidly obese, and I am no longer pre-diabetic. My list of wins is long, and all glory goes to God. My journey isn't over. I still have more weight to release, but I know that I can reach my goals through God. He wants us to "prosper and be in good health, just as your soul prospers" (3 John 1:2, NRSV).

Because of the changes in my life, and through the prompting of the Holy Spirit, I decided to become a certified health coach through *Weight Loss, God's Way* and get trained in the *Breakthrough Method*. I want to help other women who have struggled with weight throughout their lives and have given up. I want them to know that there is a better way, and that they, too, can realize their dreams of being at a healthy weight and enjoy all that comes with that. The journey may not be perfect, but it is worth it!

My Journey to Faith and Integrity

Coach Naomi Compton
MSN, RN, CRC

For as long as I can remember, being active and eating well was a part of my life. I grew up in a home where my mom made home cooked, well balanced meals every day, and my dad put my sister and me into sports at an early age. As a young adult I stayed active, but my eating habits began to change when I became more independent. I did not think much of it because I still looked fit. As a tall woman of 5'11", I could always camouflage my weight gain. Tall and slim was my look, until it wasn't.

By the time I hit my early to mid-30s, I began to experience weight gain as a result of the poor eating habits I had developed. But since I had a history of being active, I thought I knew just what to do to get this weight off. It consisted of restrictive eating and hardcore bootcamp-style workouts. For years I would be on a cycle of weight loss and gain from the distorted idea that I could just do another program to lose weight. It never crossed my mind that these programs were not sustainable. I did not even realize I was on a hamster wheel of poor health practices.

One day I found myself back at an unhealthy weight. By this time, I had started to realize restrictive programs were not very successful for me. Losing weight was not the problem. Maintaining weight loss was the issue. I had also started to experience two major setbacks to my health. First was an Achilles tendon injury I experienced in a bootcamp class. The second was the turmoil of excessive bleeding and iron deficiency anemia I was experiencing as a result of the multiple fibroid tumors growing around my uterus. As crazy as it sounds, I am now thankful for these health issues because without them I may not have realized the need for change.

By the way, did I mention I am a registered nurse (RN)? I have been an RN for over 22 years. Throughout many of those years, and in conjunction with the experiences I have shared so far, I was also dealing with the internal conflict of being a healthcare professional with an unhealthy lifestyle. This internal conflict felt like a billboard hovering over me displaying my lack of integrity. But out of fear, I never felt inclined to speak about it or address it. The turning point of my health journey occurred while studying the Breakthrough Principle of Courage.

As a child, I had a fear of EVERYTHING! A fear of dogs, people, drowning, the Easter Bunny. You name it, I was probably scared of it. Though many of those fears had been addressed over my life, what had not been addressed was my awareness of how fear took precedence over my faith and prevented me from moving forward. The Breakthrough Principle of Courage (Principle #12) helped me understand that the goal isn't to not be afraid but to identify the fears and be transformed so that God fulfills my needs. God would begin to transform my fear of the unknown, of judgment, and of rejection into experiences He would use in my faith journey.

As I began to offer my body as a living sacrifice and be transformed and renewed (Romans 12:1-2), I became aware of the many burdens I placed on myself. I was in the process of unlearning and relearning. I prayed God would soften my heart and open my mind to what He wanted me to take away. As a fitness enthusiast/former instructor and a registered nurse, I had a lot of knowledge. God showed me that I had been learning but not coming to knowledge of the Truth (2 Timothy 3:7). As God continues to transform me, He has made me aware of the fact that transparency leads to transformation. He has transformed me to look at Him as my source instead of looking at myself as the source. The more vulnerable and transparent I am with God and with the people in the community He has placed me in, the more I begin to experience transformation in my mind and my body. I continue to lose weight sustainably, having dumped the hamster wheel of obsession and despair.

Now I am navigating a life of freedom through releasing, retaining, and receiving.

Release: I began to let go of trying to control the scale through unsustainable lifestyle practices. I began to let go of the idea that there was a perfect situation that needed to occur in order for me to make the faith move in becoming a health coach. I began to let go of the "sneaky pride" I had been experiencing. I define sneaky pride as giving into those feelings of insufficiency that lead to the lie that I am not good enough even when God has called me to something. This becomes prideful because, essentially, I am asserting my will above God's. It is sneaky because, on the surface, it does not look like pride, but it certainly is. I also began to release behaviors that were no longer serving me. The main one being alcohol consumption. As a mixologist and herbal nurse, creating and blending are activities I really enjoy. One day I realized I no longer wanted to mix or drink alcoholic beverages. I would focus on the teas I loved to make. This has proven to be a bigger blessing than I could have imagined, and something I never intended on doing.

Retain: I began to recognize the practices in my life that were beneficial and should stay. Practices such as intimacy with God, my love for fitness and nutritious meals, my enjoyment of nature. These practices grew to become even more valuable to me. God began to increase my capacity and love for these and more. I became more intentional with what God allowed me to retain. As a result, I am witnessing how this intentionality is impacting those around me.

Receive: God's grace has shown up abundantly in my life. Receiving does not always have to be tangible, but it might be. One of the major gifts I received from God was clarity in my vision of connecting my occupation as a RN with my vocation as a Christian Health Coach. It is in the intimate moments with Him that my confidence in my calling continues to grow. At an early age, I was taught by my parents that my spiritual gifts and talents are not for myself but to share with others. I am now committed to walking alongside other Christian nurses and women seeking freedom, integrity, and breakthroughs in their health.

My Journey of Resilience and Transformation

Coach Monique Feast

My journey towards health began a year after the birth of my second daughter. Weight was never an issue for me. I used to be the person who could eat when and how I wanted, then go to sleep afterwards. However, during and after the birth of my second daughter, I was at my highest weight I had ever been in my life.

Little did I know this was the beginning of my health and weight release journey. I tried two different diet plans at that time. One was Weight Watchers, but that didn't work for me. The other was Isagenix and I experienced great success following this program. I lost 17 pounds the first month and 10 pounds the second month. I started at 172 pounds and I finished at 145 pounds. I went from a size 14/16 to a 6/8. I was able to maintain my weight for years.

In my late forties I started experiencing perimenopause and switched to a vegan diet. When I turned 49 I began the Keto diet because I wanted to be at a certain weight for my 50th birthday. I did achieve my goal. However, my perimenopause symptoms became excruciating and I was experiencing severe hot flashes, about 20 to 25 a day with and/or without heart palpitations; sometimes I did not even realize I was sweating. I was anxious. Panic attacks would happen out of nowhere. Crying spells, too. I had low energy, headaches, digestive issues, mood swings and, of course, weight gain especially around my midsection. Oh, did I mention that I was still healing from a past trauma that seemed to join the party of afflicting my mind, body, and soul? I was a hormonal hot mess. Needless to say at 50 I was told I was post-menopausal and my doctor applauded me for going through the process naturally but advised me to get on HRT. I did and it helped with the hot flashes and some of the other symptoms.

Now I had some physical relief of menopause, but not mental relief. This led me on a journey to seek greater understanding of how my hormones affected me in the season of menopause. I was in a stage of wrestling and struggling spiritually, mentally, and physically. Physically, I was suffering. Sometimes my symptoms were so debilitating all I could do was go to bed. I felt like I was losing myself, let alone losing my mind. I honestly did not like myself or the woman I saw in the mirror. I looked like I was six- months' pregnant. I was not able to put on my clothes without my friend Spanx. I wasn't pregnant with a child but with a lot of visceral fat that became stored around my organs due to insulin resistance and inflammation in my body. Mentally, I had negative and toxic thoughts that were so ingrained on a subconscious level that they affected me on a conscious level. Some of those thoughts were: "I am not worthy", "I am not enough", "Something must be wrong with me", "I need that person to love, accept or validate me". I was riddled with shame and guilt, seeking the approval of others, and lack of forgiveness for myself. Through my searching, I came across a challenge from *Weight Loss, God's Way*. I joined the challenge and learned about the Breakthrough Principles. Little did I know that the principles in the *Breakthrough Method* would serve as a catalyst on my journey of health and healing. As I opened my heart to learning and applying the principles in *Weight Loss, God's Way* I had to be honest with God and myself.

Shame, insecurity, depression, PTSD, anxiety, and grief were constant companions of mine. The horrific experiences of sexual trauma, the death of my mom when I was 16, a rocky relationship with my father, then his death, and flunking out of college to work two and three jobs just to support myself depleted me spiritually, mentally, and physically. I was lost and needed help. I suppressed, rationalized, and denied my feelings through food, partying, and unhealthy relationships in the hope of being validated and loved.

Applying the principles of renewing my mind, stewarding the temple God has entrusted to me, and accepting that I am redeemed from my past are gifts from my God.

I understand that I have not experienced anything new that another woman has not experienced, but from my experience it is a story of hope, redemption, and healing. From my story I desire to empower, encourage, support, and challenge women through their own hormonal journeys of pre-, peri-, and post-menopause that have those last 5 to 50 pounds of weight to release spiritually, mentally, and/or physically. I look forward to applying Hebrews 12:1-2.

> "Therefore we also, since we are surrounded by so great a cloud of witnesses, let us lay aside every weight, and the sin which so easily ensnares us, and let us run with endurance the race that is set before us, looking unto Jesus, the author and finisher of our faith, who for the joy that was set before Him endured the cross, despising the shame, and has sat down at the right hand of the throne of God".

My Journey to Renewing My Mind

Coach Lynette Gee

I've found my voice, breaking free from the shackles of the facade I've worn for so long. In a moment of raw honesty, I acknowledged a daunting truth—I had been living behind a mask. The words I uttered aloud resonated deep within: *'Everyone is living their best life, but me.'* It was a stark realization, a reflection of a mindset far removed from the grace and compassion of Christ that I strive to embody.

I am Lynette Gee, a coach's wife for over 33 years, blessed with three biological children and two more bestowed upon me by God's grace. Our journey, marked by countless relocations due to my husband's career in college coaching, unveiled a pattern of unhealthy self-neglect. My focus was unwaveringly fixed on ensuring the safety, security, and prosperity of my family, but in the process I lost sight of my own needs and aspirations for thriving.

As we moved from city to city, tirelessly establishing homes, schools, and support systems for my family, I inadvertently left myself behind. Somewhere along this dedicated path, seeds of jealousy and resentment began to sprout within me, aimed not at others but at the very family I so dearly loved. I found myself envious of their flourishing lives. It was a harrowing revelation to resent the efforts that were meant to foster their growth. Although I continued to do those things for my family, the way I served was deeply influenced by my negative attitude.

Exhausted and emotionally burdened, I sought solace in food and television, attempting to fill the void of loneliness that seemed to engulf me amidst the silence of new surroundings. My emotional journey with overeating has been a rollercoaster ride. It's not just about consuming excessive amounts of food. It's a complex interplay of emotions, thoughts, and habits.

There are moments of comfort and solace in food. When life gets tough, it's easy to turn to familiar flavors and textures for a sense of relief. The act of eating can provide a temporary escape from stress, sadness, or even boredom. It's like a warm, comforting embrace during challenging times.

However, this emotional journey also has its dark side. Overeating often leads to guilt, shame, and self-criticism. Those moments of indulgence can quickly turn into regret as I grapple with the consequences. The weight gain, the feeling of loss of control, and the knowledge that I'm not taking care of myself all weigh heavily on my mind.

It's a cycle that's hard to break. The emotional highs and lows of overeating become a familiar pattern, making it challenging to adopt healthier habits. But I'm on a journey of self-discovery and self-improvement, seeking to understand the root causes of my emotional eating and finding healthier ways to cope with life's ups and downs. It's a journey of self-compassion, learning to forgive myself for past mistakes and gradually finding balance in my relationship with food and emotions. In this struggle, God led me to *Weight Loss, God's Way*. Initially, I attributed my weight gain to various external factors, but through this transformative journey I began to delve deeper, understanding the emotional roots of my struggles.

God used this weight gain as a beacon, guiding me to explore my true identity in Him. I learned to discern the false narratives and emotions that were holding me captive, to recognize the seasons of resentment as moments of fear and loneliness. Through this program and others like Positive Intelligence®, I embarked on a path of growth, both spiritually and mentally.

I remember reading Romans 12:2 and thinking, "God, I need You to renew my mind, because unless I do I won't recognize Your good, pleasing, and perfect will." Romans 12:2 is indeed a powerful verse that highlights the need for a renewed mind in order to discern God's good, pleasing, and perfect will. It's a beautiful acknowledgment of our dependence on God's transformative work in our lives to align our thoughts and desires with His divine purpose.

As I journeyed through this process, something remarkable happened—I started to thrive. My physical health improved, my stress levels decreased, and my overall outlook on life became more positive. But what was even more significant was the profound shift in my perspective.

I became grateful, for I had come to realize that God used my weight gain to draw me closer to Him. Through this journey I embraced my true self in Christ, shattering the chains of negativity and lies that once bound me. I learned to pause and redirect the negative thoughts, embracing the liberating truth of God's word that defines who I truly am.

I also began to see the incredible potential for transformation within each of us. I realized that my own journey, though difficult, had equipped me with the knowledge and empathy to guide others on their paths to wellness.

It was at this point that I felt a calling to become a wellness coach and share the wisdom I had gained through my own experiences. I wanted to help others navigate their own challenges and discover their inner strength. I knew that wellness was not just about physical health but also about nurturing the mind, body, and spirit.

Becoming a wellness coach was not a decision I took lightly. It required training, education, and a commitment to ongoing personal growth. But every step of the way felt purposeful and fulfilling. I gained the tools and knowledge needed to support others on their wellness journeys, and felt a profound sense of fulfillment in doing so.

Today, as a wellness coach, I am deeply inspired by the individuals I have the privilege to work with. I've witnessed incredible transformations—people overcoming obstacles, reclaiming their health, and embracing life with newfound vigor. My journey from struggle to wellness coach is a reminder that our challenges can be our greatest teachers, and our experiences can be used to inspire and empower others.

I am grateful for the path I have walked, and I am dedicated to helping others, be it my fellow coach wives or anyone who struggles with their weight, to discover their own paths to wellness, resilience, and fulfillment. It is a calling that brings me immense joy and purpose, and I am excited to continue this journey of transformation alongside those I have the honor of coaching.

My Journey to Freedom: Breaking the Bonds of Control and Perfectionism

Coach Laura Foster

My initial struggles with excess weight began after giving birth to my son. It was by trial and error that I gained and lost weight. Choosing what to eat and how much to eat was not a pleasant experience. None of the solutions to weight loss provided REAL, lasting solutions for me, and I tried many over the years.

After years of yo-yo dieting, gaining more weight, being diagnosed as pre-diabetic, and getting emotionally exhausted, I realized that I could not win this battle on my own. I earnestly cried out to the Lord for help. I mean I cried real tears as I prayed and asked for His help. I was at the end of my rope and had to let go and let God.

God led me to a devotional by Cathy Morenzie on my Bible app.

For the first time, I was given a Spirit-led, faith-centered weight loss plan that fostered a deeper relationship with God. This was a challenge for me because I had to relinquish control and submit my will to God. How did I do it? I'm glad you asked. It didn't happen immediately. I was kicking and screaming and outright rebellious. Accustomed to my independence and doing things my way when it came to choosing what to eat and when to exercise, it was difficult to relinquish the reins to God. After all, I'm a grown-up. However, God who is patient, merciful, understanding, and loving saw through my pain and rebellion. He didn't abandon me. He knew my reasons, struggles, and fears were driving my bad behavior.

As I began reading the devotional, *Healthy by Design: Weight Loss, God's Way*, I knew in my heart that God had answered my cry for help. After going through the seven-day devotional, I became a member of *Weight Loss, God's Way* and began taking the courses. Every principle each course addressed aligned with the Word of God. God was speaking to me through the courses; guiding me, teaching me, and revealing the lies and wrong thinking I believed for years.

I was slowly changing my negative thoughts to Godly thoughts. I spoke what God said about me to myself until I believed it. I regained my self-esteem and confidence with each pound I released.

During a *Weight Loss, God's Way* coaching session, I discovered the principle of Overcoming Emotional Eating. This marked a turning point in my life. I realized that my thoughts of "I deserve" and "It's not fair" were contributing to my emotional eating and weight gain. With a new sense of purpose and ever-increasing faith, I relinquished control over my journey and entrusted it to God.

My approach to nutrition, exercise, and self-care with a faith-driven mindset emerged when I joined the *Weight Loss, God's Way* online program. Previously, meal planning had been absent from my life for some time. Exercise was not robust. Self-care with a faith-driven mindset took a backseat on my list of priorities. Everything was restored after becoming a *Weight Loss, God's Way* member.

Still, my struggles with control and perfectionism in my weight loss journey kept me in bondage. When the progress was too slow to my liking, I went back to doing it my way. When I stepped outside my boundaries, I replaced self-compassion with self-criticism. Stirring up my faith, I submitted everything to God and committed to speaking affirmations of God's truths over myself.

The transformative power of surrendering my goals to God's timing and plan has freed me from anxiety, sleepless nights, and a fear of failure. God never fails, worries, or slumbers. As I moved toward health and wellness, I discerned that my journey, faith, and the transformative power of the Breakthrough Principles that Cathy Morenzie teaches is meant to be shared with other women struggling to be set free.

My impact on my family and community as they witness my transformation is humbling and gratifying. They see God's hand on my life and are encouraged that God is no respecter of persons. If He did it for me, He will do it for them.

My triumphant moment of reaching my healthy goal weight will be praising and glorifying God for His faithfulness, celebrating with my son, daughter-in-law, and grandchildren, and living free of debilitating diseases and medications.

Today I stand as a light on a hill for others to see how God responds to prayers of faith and His word, through the Breakthrough Method outlined in this book.

My story is a testimony of God's power, goodness, love, and faithfulness toward me and His people. Through sharing my journey I hope to inspire others to deepen their faith, embrace the transformative power of the Breakthrough Method, and trust God to do what He's promised.

My Journey to Healing: Overcoming Emotional Eating

Coach Shannon Kay McCoy

Growing up, I had always enjoyed good health and a physically active lifestyle. Engaged in cheerleading and track during high school, I was a petite and fit young woman. Life was relatively smooth until I crossed paths with the man who would later become my husband. Initially, I believed he shared my faith, but over time it became evident that it was all mere words. Our marriage took a significant turn for the worse, and I found myself confronted with challenges I had never encountered before.

As my faith continued to grow, I began to see the devastating impact of deception in my marriage. This phase marked the most challenging period of my life, turning my world upside down. My finances were in disarray, my life was veering off track, and I descended into a deep state of depression. In the depths of my despair, I sought solace in the familiar comforts of late-night eating and the mind-numbing refuge of binge-watching television. The reality I faced had become too harsh to bear, and I desperately needed an escape from the overwhelming negative emotions that threatened to engulf me. I couldn't bring myself to confront these emotions head-on, and thus I unwittingly turned to food as my refuge, my confidant, and my escape.

It was a dangerous pattern that unfolded, a rhythm dictated by my emotions. When sadness cast its heavy shadow over my heart, I sought solace in the temporary comfort of food. Food became a reliable companion in my moments of sorrow, a source of fleeting joy that, while short-lived, offered a respite from the pain that threatened to overwhelm me.

In moments of profound emotional pain I found myself reaching for snacks and indulging in mindless eating, filling the void with flavors and textures that momentarily distracted me from the demise of my life. The act of eating became a ritual, a way to pass the time and briefly escape the clutches of despair. Food, in those instances, served as a form of emotional comfort, a diversion from the feelings of emptiness that enveloped me.

When anger raged within, food became my outlet for venting the pent-up frustration that boiled just beneath the surface. Each bite was a release, a way to channel my emotions into something tangible if only for a moment. The act of eating during these times was almost cathartic, a means of expression when words failed to convey the intensity of my feelings.

And in moments of sheer exhaustion and fatigue food was my crutch, my source of quick energy, and a fleeting escape from the demands of a tiring day. The sugary or savory delights I consumed provided a momentary surge of vitality, a brief respite from the relentless weariness that threatened to consume me.

This unhealthy coping mechanism, though temporarily comforting, ultimately perpetuated a destructive cycle. It offered momentary relief but left me trapped in a never-ending loop of overindulgence, followed by guilt and self-loathing. I had unwittingly created an unhealthy relationship with food, using it to escape my emotions rather than facing them. It took time, support, and a renewed sense of faith to break free from this cycle and find healthier ways to address the emotional challenges I faced.

I felt like a stranger in my own skin, hiding behind baggy clothes and eyeglasses. Depression led to isolation as I withdrew from social activities, limiting my interactions primarily to attending church and work. On a spiritual level, I grappled with reconciling my faith with my ongoing battle against overeating. I attempted various diets, weight loss programs and exercise regimens, but nothing seemed to provide a lasting solution. I was ensnared in a vicious cycle of overeating, misery, shame, and guilt.

It was only when I stumbled upon scriptures that shed light on the sin of gluttony that I started to grasp the gravity of my situation. Proverbs 23:21's warning, "For the heavy drinker and the glutton will come to poverty," hit close to home. Philippians 3:18-19 painted a grim picture of those controlled by their appetites. These verses made me uncomfortable, but I still wasn't fully convicted of my sin.

Seeking divine guidance, I prayed fervently for the conviction I couldn't muster on my own because I was a true food addict, resistant to letting go of my addiction. In a testament to God's love and faithfulness, my prayer was answered, and I began to feel the conviction necessary to embark on the path of repentance for my gluttony. This transformation didn't occur overnight; it involved a gradual process of self-awareness, renewing my mind and changing my mindset.

The Breakthrough Principles became my bedrock, fortifying my commitment to overcoming emotional eating and mastering my mindset. They provided me with the essential frameworks to remain on the path of recovery, offering ongoing accountability.

These principles not only defined the nature of my struggle but also illuminated the way out, offering a clear and well-structured approach to address the complex issues of emotional eating and mental strongholds.

Emotional eating, I realized, was not just about food; it was a coping mechanism I had unknowingly adopted to navigate the turbulent waters of my emotions. The Breakthrough Principles guided me in understanding the root causes of my emotional eating patterns, helping me uncover the triggers and emotions that drove me to seek solace in food. It was a process of self-discovery, of peeling back the layers of my own psyche to reveal the intricate connections between my feelings and my eating habits.

Furthermore, these principles equipped me with invaluable tools for mastering my mindset. Emotional eating was not just a physical habit; it was deeply intertwined with my thought patterns and beliefs about food, self-worth, and coping with emotions. Through the Breakthrough Principles I learned to reframe my mindset, to challenge and change the negative thought patterns that perpetuated emotional eating. This transformation of my mental landscape was a crucial aspect of my journey to freedom.

The ongoing accountability offered by these principles was like a steady hand guiding me along the path to recovery. It was a support system that ensured

I stayed on course, even during moments of temptation or weakness. The principles served as a source of strength when my own resolve wavered, reminding me of the ultimate goal of overall health and well-being that I was working towards.

By sharing my story I aim to inspire and encourage women who, like me, have grappled with emotional eating. I want them to know that there is hope and a way to break free from the cycle of using food as a crutch for their emotions.

I share my story because I am committed to instilling hope and support women who grapple with emotional eating. I want them to understand that it is possible to conquer this struggle and attain the health goals that God has intended for them. Through faith in and a commitment to heal, I found freedom from emotional eating, and I firmly believe that others can do the same.

My Journey of Transformation, Empowerment, and Faith

Coach Debbie Lehman

Welcome to the first day of the rest of your life! My name is Debbie Lehman, and I've embarked on a truly transformative journey, shedding over 150 pounds after discovering the inspiring Christian program, *Weight Loss, God's Way*. For most of my adult life, I grappled with the relentless challenge of weight management. I tried countless weight loss approaches, but they only brought fleeting success, and the weight always returned, as if it had a magnetic pull, like a lifelong companion.

It was difficult to escape the clutches of obesity, and I had reluctantly accepted a life burdened with pain and fraught with unhealthy circumstances, weighing over 350 pounds. This was not the life I had envisioned for myself.

My relationship with God had always been present in my life. I had given my heart to the Lord at the tender age of thirteen. However, for the most part, I kept Jesus tucked away in my back pocket, reserved for the most challenging and turbulent times. It hadn't occurred to me then that He cares about even the most seemingly insignificant moments of our lives. It was a revelation waiting to happen.

At the same time, I believed that my purpose revolved around being a devoted wife and a dedicated mother to my three sons. Their well-being was my top priority, and my personal needs took a back seat, buried beneath layers of responsibilities and obligations. I dedicated myself wholeheartedly to nurturing their growth and development, and I cherished every moment of motherhood. Yet, amidst all this love and care, I had overlooked my own needs.

Then came the day when my sons had flown the nest and were busy raising their own families. I found myself at a crossroads, staring at an empty nest and a reflection in the mirror that bore the physical and emotional scars of years of self-neglect. I turned my attention to my career and dedicated myself to volunteer work, channeling my energies into these endeavors. Once again, I allowed my own health and well-being to take a back seat to other facets of my life.

On the surface, I projected an image of a happy and successful person, but on the inside, I was grappling with an overpowering sense of misery. The void was growing, and I couldn't ignore it any longer.

Then, in the summer of 2021, a ray of hope entered my life. I was reading my daily devotion on the Bible app when I noticed an advertisement for something called *Weight Loss, God's Way*. My curiosity piqued, I followed the link and decided to participate in a challenge they were offering. From the very beginning, I felt a deep connection to the program. It was as if Cathy Morenzie, the program's creator, was speaking directly to me through her words and guidance. This was something truly special, and I could sense it in every fiber of my being.

The challenge was like a small taste of something extraordinary, and I knew I had to delve deeper. I eagerly signed up for a three-month program, and that's when the real transformation began.

Weight Loss, God's Way was not just a diet plan; it was a holistic program that integrated faith, inspiration, and empowerment into the journey of weight loss. Cathy Morenzie's guidance wasn't just about the numbers on the scale but about nurturing the body, mind, and spirit. It was a comprehensive approach that made me realize the power of faith in achieving my goals.

The program encouraged me to reconnect with my faith, to bring Jesus out of the back pocket and into every aspect of my life, especially the journey of weight loss. I discovered that faith could provide the strength and resolve to overcome even the most daunting challenges.

One of the fundamental principles of *Weight Loss, God's Way* was setting realistic and sustainable goals. It wasn't about losing weight as fast as possible; it was about making lasting changes. Gradual, steady progress became my mantra. I embraced a balanced diet, incorporating more fruits, vegetables, lean proteins, and whole grains while consciously limiting processed foods and refined sugars. Portion control became my ally.

Exercise took on a new meaning in my life. It wasn't a chore; it was a joyful activity that I incorporated into my daily routine. I discovered activities that I loved, whether it was riding my stationary bike, enrolling in line dance classes or taking walks with my husband. The key was consistency, and I made exercise an integral part of my life.

But *Weight Loss, God's Way* went beyond the physical. It delved into the emotional aspects of weight management. Stress and emotional eating had always been my pitfalls. The program provided tools to address these challenges enabling me to overcome them. It emphasized the importance of quality sleep, which had a profound impact on my overall well-being.

A significant part of my journey was seeking support from friends, family, and the community. It was reassuring to know that I wasn't alone in this endeavor. *Weight Loss, God's Way* fostered a sense of togetherness and support that propelled me forward.

As the days turned into weeks and the weeks into months, I saw the pounds melt away. It was not always easy, but with the Lord's amazing grace, coupled with the knowledge and tools provided by the program, kept me on track. The feeling of empowerment grew, and I became an inspiration to others, proving that lasting change was not only possible but achievable with dedication, faith, and the right guidance.

My journey was not just about shedding pounds; it was a holistic transformation towards a healthier, happier life. *Weight Loss, God's Way* was not just a program; it was a beacon of hope, guiding me towards sustainable success. As the weight steadily decreased, my inner peace and self-esteem soared. I had discovered the path to a brighter future, and I couldn't be more grateful for the day I clicked on that advertisement.

In retrospect, my story is a testament to the power of faith, inspiration, and empowerment in achieving success. It's proof that if we keep our focus on the Lord, we can overcome even the most challenging circumstances and rewrite the narrative of our lives. Today, I am a living example that it's never too late to prioritize self-care, embrace change, and find peace through faith and inspiration.

The journey of weight loss is not just about shedding pounds; it's about discovering a healthier, happier version of oneself. And I'm here to say that it's possible, and it's worth every step of the way. My *Weight Loss, God's Way* journey is living proof that if at 70 years old I can do this, YOU can too.

In closing, my transformation journey through *Weight Loss, God's Way* has not only changed my life but has inspired me to become a certified health coach. I am passionate about guiding and supporting others in their own journeys towards a healthier, more fulfilling life. If you're ready to take the first step towards achieving your goals, both physically and spiritually, I am here to walk with you on this path of transformation. Together, we can discover the incredible strength and grace that faith and wellness can bring into our lives. Your journey can start today, and I look forward to being a part of it.

My Journey: Surrendering to God's Will and Finding Hope

Coach Julie Spezzano

I was done. I was at my breaking point. I had given my last ounce of patience and my last ray of hope. Have you ever been there? I had three daughters and didn't see any hope or value to pass on. I was so lost; I no longer knew who was looking back at me in the mirror. Who was she? What do I have to offer my children? **Ezra 8:21** *says that we might humble ourselves before our God and ask Him for a safe journey for us and our children.* I wasn't just asking, I was begging! I knew I was ready. I was ready to battle and find the woman within. To find some sense of wholeness to pass on to my girls. To create a legacy for them to be proud of and to carry on.

Oh, but the giants that were in my way! Growing up, I never had healthy emotional encouragement or support. My dad struggled with alcohol and my mom did the best she could, but was fearful of making things worse. She had her own battle with self- confidence, value, and worth. So, yes, food was our choice. It was legal and safe. Or so we thought! It wasn't long before we used ice cream and popcorn as rewards on the nights that our emotions were running high. Yep, the trap was set, and the bait was there. Addiction had reared its ugly head and ensnared us to think we were in control. For years I hid it well, and was active enough to hide the pounds.

I guess I thought it wouldn't change. I could hide it forever. After the birth of my second child, I learned otherwise. My weight afterwards was even higher, and it didn't come off as easily as before. I had as many different excuses as I did pounds. Both were weighing me down. Now was the time to tackle my weight head-on and show everyone what I could do. But my past failures had other plans. Once again it had raised its ugly head and attacked! Grabbing me before I could even begin to fight. Trapped, stuck, and frozen with fear, I was unable to break through, to find a way out. I stayed that way for 20 years. My kids grew up, left home, and started their own families.

I just couldn't give up! I couldn't give in! Or could I? Can you?

That was the moment, my turnaround. I knew I had to find a way. I was losing faith in myself and hope in my journey. I had been around this mountain before. I had climbed to the top and "lost the weight", but before I could celebrate… I stumbled, fell, and came crashing down the hill once again. You know that feeling when you've just had enough? You're tired of the backaches, the tight clothes, and wondering if the is any chance at all that the weight will come off? I was defeated and broken. I knew it was time.

Matt. 11:28-30 rang in my ears. *"Come to me all you who are weary and burdened, and I will give you rest. Take my yoke upon you and learn from me, for I am gentle and humble in heart. I will find rest for your souls. For my yoke is easy and my burden is light."* But is there a way to still hope, or even a chance?

There is! Your very first step was picking up this book! You are ready. Remember when I said I didn't want to give in? It was the best choice I ever made. I chose to surrender my will for God's will. You can too! *Weight Loss, God's Way* has a proven method to get the weight off. Even better than that, you will learn how to keep it off. No gross foods or massive restrictions! You choose the path to take. It's your journey. The lesson plans along the way will create in you a willingness to see yourself from the inside, through the looking glass, and eventually even in the mirror. You will not only see health as your new identity. You will discover new ways to make your life whole again. With a total body, mind, and spirit connection. Yes, it will take some work and dedication, but close your eyes and envision your deepest dream. Now look up, I'm here to help you.

Just imagine the thrill of surviving the battle. Wait! Better yet, going from survivor to thriver! WLGW will take you on that journey! I would love to walk beside you. Through the fear, self-doubt, and temptations you've struggled with in the past. To help you discover and understand your God-given assignment and share your story with others. (Yes, you have one!) To pass on faith and hope to those still struggling. Creating your own new legacy. Your own new identity in Christ. Breakthrough from just surviving to thriving. You've got this!

Metamorphosis: The Lifelong Transformative Journey of My Mind, Body, and Soul

Coach Monica L. Holloway, LPC, NCC, CHC

On December 26, 1979, I was born into my family and life outside of the womb began. Much like a butterfly egg is placed on a plant, I was strategically placed by God into my environment which would become the place where I would learn, grow, and receive nourishment. As a baby I was unable to feed myself and relied solely on my parents to ensure that I was receiving adequate food and drink. Being that my parents are from the South, growing up, the food I became accustomed to was "soul food". Macaroni and cheese, collard greens, yams, cornbread, pound cake, sweet tea, and the list goes on. Anything you can consider "soul food", trust and believe I received it and loved it for breakfast, lunch, and dinner. Healthy eating and getting active were not something that was ever mentioned, discussed, or modeled, and eating was often the main event when family would come together for holidays, birthdays, funerals, family reunions, and Sunday dinners after church. Over the years I would continue to indulge in emotional eating when I was happy or sad (unintentionally learned behaviors) and not regularly move my body, and it took me to a place of depression, fatigue, and low self-esteem. At my worst point I did not realize that was my best point as it prompted me into action. Although I could not see it at that moment, my future was showing.

During the feeding stage of life, a caterpillar's sole purpose is to eat food and grow to move forward in the next phase of its purpose. Over my years of life, I had learned how to "feed" my body, but never how to truly nourish or fuel it. I had also learned how to "feed" my mind negative thoughts about myself due to being overweight. I would fill my body with junk and wonder why often I would feel fatigued or depleted. I would go through this cycle numerous times and try almost every single pill or exercise program that would come on TV. The first of every month became my "start over date" for my latest and greatest weight loss endeavor. I knew I had become desperate when I started to inject myself with liraglutide to suppress my appetite, when I hate needles and pain. It got to the point where I could not button or tie my shoe without being out of breath because my stomach was so big. I went to a theme park and was embarrassed because I could not get the harness to buckle. I was on a plane and could barely buckle my seatbelt and/or fit into the seat. It got to the point when I looked in the mirror I would not truly "look" at myself because I did not like what was staring back at me and who I had become, and it was affecting my ability to embrace my identity in Christ. Enough had become enough, and I was truly sick and tired of being sick and tired. I was ready for a change.

I was truly in a place of darkness and could not see my way out alone. I prayed to God to help me to get through this and to be a healthier version of myself. During this time my relationship with God was increasing as well as my ability to eat healthier, exercise more, and get my mind right (literally). At the time I was a part of a bible study with a women's group, and it was just what was needed to encourage, inspire, and uplift me during that time. God will place the right people in your life at the right time to help you get through those hard times. It was during this time that I realized there are no quick fixes, and that releasing weight will take discipline and commitment and nothing less. I had to do a serious values check to get some things in order and work on prioritizing and time management. Over the last year I have released 70 pounds and numerous inches, and have truly learned the importance of fueling my body, mind, and spirit with the right things.

In my role of a Licensed Professional Counselor, I tell my clients often that the things that we go through are never just about us. The very things that we struggle with the most are the areas that God wants us to be able to share with others as a source of encouragement and inspiration. I have not mastered healthy eating and exercise by any means, but I am constantly becoming better and growing in my ability to continue to establish discipline and consistency. I continue daily to work towards overcoming emotional eating, mindset mastery, and having the courage to move forward with my health goals. My breaking point was my "waking" point, and allowed me to see so clearly how helping others with holistic health as a Christian Health Coach is connected to my purpose.

During my Peer-To-Peer Coach Certification Weekend with *Weight Loss, God's Way*, I received confirmation that I was moving in the right direction with pursuing my Christian Health Coach Certification. As I went through the curriculum of *The Breakthrough Method*, I experienced some of the very breakthroughs that I am excited for my clients to experience as well. I submit this gift and privilege of being a health coach to God and am committed to lifelong development to help others in their holistic health journeys. I will leave you with this scripture, as it is so important for us to realize that our whole being belongs to God—Body, Mind, and Soul—and we must ensure we are "fueling" all of them with the right things for holistic health.

> **1 Corinthians 6:19-20 (MSG)** *"Or didn't you realize that your body is a sacred place, the place of the Holy Spirit? Don't you see that you can't live however you please, squandering what God paid such a high price for? The physical part of you is not some piece of property belonging to the spiritual part of you. God owns the whole works."*

Next Steps

Can I get an amen for those powerful shares and testimonies! Truly inspiring on multiple levels.

As we come to the end of this incredible journey through the stories of our eleven exceptional coaches, I'm filled with gratitude for the wisdom, strength, and inspiration they have shared. The lessons and insights shared by our coaches serve as a guide, lighting the way forward for those of you who seek real life answers from real life women.

I want to express my heartfelt appreciation to our coaches for their openness, honesty, and unwavering commitment to serving others. Their stories will continue to inspire, offering hope and guidance to others on their own paths to health. Together, we can break free from the shackles of unhealthy habits and discover the joy of living a life that truly glorifies God. The harvest is plenty and the workers are few, but God has raised these mighty women to serve in His kingdom as health ambassadors.

As you close this book and move forward on your personal journey, remember that you are not alone. Our coaches are here to support and guide you, and you have a community of individuals who share your goals and aspirations.

Take the next step on your journey with a complimentary coaching session with one of our skilled coaches:

weightlossgodswaycoaches.com

Thank You

Thank you for being motivated, courageous, inquisitive, and committed to go deeper in your health journey and uncover the missing piece— Christ!

I pray that these principles have been as much of a blessing to you as they have been for me and the hundreds of thousands of women around the world who have experienced what it means to include God in their health and weight-releasing journey.

If you've been blessed by this book, then please don't keep it a secret!

There are millions of women who need to hear this message. Please take a moment to leave an honest book review so more people can discover this book as well.

This book has laid out a great foundation for you, but there's so much more for you to discover. Please keep in touch with me so that you can stay in this conversation and continue to make your health a priority —God's Way. Plus I'll send you a free copy of my '3 Steps to Overcome Emotional Eating' guide when you enroll for my weekly devotional message on successful weight loss, God's way.

Receive my weekly posts at CathyMorenzie.com

Other books by Cathy Morenzie

Weight Loss, God's Way:
The Proven 21-Day Weight Loss
Devotional

Weight Loss, God's Way:
Low-Carb Cookbook and Meal-Plan

Healthy Eating, God's Way

Get Active, God's Way

Spirit-Filled & Sugar-Free

Pray Powerfully, Lose Weight

Love God, Lose Weight

The Word on Weight Loss

Available at:
ChristianWeightLossBooks.com
And your favorite place to buy books

Christian Weight Loss Books and Programs

Weight Loss, God's Way equips women to rely on God as their strength so they can live in freedom, joy, and peace. At the end of the day, that's what we really want. Let's be honest, if you never achieved that mythical, elusive number on the scale, but were fully able to live a life of freedom, joy, and peace, would that be enough? I know for me the answer is a resounding 'YES!!!'

We provide a multidimensional approach to releasing weight. It encompasses the whole person—spiritual, psychological, mental, nutritional, physical, and even hormonal! We believe that you must address the whole person — body, soul, and spirit. If you're looking for a program that just tells you what to eat and what exercises to do, this ain't it.

This program has helped thousands of women break free from all the roadblocks that have been hindering their weight loss success while discovering their identity in Christ.

The Weight Loss, God's Way Program offers a variety of free and paid courses and programs.

They include the following:

A YouVersion Bible Study

A free basic introduction to Step 1 of the Weight Loss, God's Way program. To learn more, go to:

https://www.bible.com/reading-plans/20974-weight-lossgods-way-cathy-morenzie

Or from the YouVersion Bible App, click the bottom center, 'check-mark' button to open devotions, and search for 'Healthy by Design to find our free devotionals.

The Weight Loss, God's Way Newsletter

Join the free Weight Loss, God's Way community and receive weekly posts designed to help you align your weight loss with God's Word. You'll also receive our '70 Simple and Powerful Tips You can Start Immediately to Lose Weight' guide free. To join the newsletter, sign up at:

cathymorenzie.com

The Membership Program

A done-for-you, step-by-step guide to the entire program. We lead our members through a different weight loss devotional every month tackling subjects from emotional eating, prayer, self-esteem to workouts and (of course) healthy eating. Dozens of bonus tools like group coaching calls, forums, and accountability groups are available. To become a Weight Loss, God's Way member, go to:

weightlossgodsway.com

Bible Studies for Churches and Small Groups

The membership program can also be experienced a la carte with a group of your friends or with your church. Take one of our three- to-six-week studies on a variety of health and weight-releasing topics. To learn more about starting a Bible study in your home or church, go to:

https://www.cathymorenzie.com/start-a-wlgw-group/

Books and Devotionals

You can find all of our Healthy by Design series of weight loss books here:

christianweightlossbooks.com

Keynote Speaking

Want me to visit your hometown? Need a speaker for your annual conference or special event? My fun and practical approach to Weight Loss, God's

Way will give your group clarity and focus to move toward their weight loss goals. To learn more or to book a speaking engagement, visit:

https://www.cathymorenzie.com/speaking/

Private Coaching

Prefer a more one-on-one approach? I have a few dedicated time slots available to coach you individually to help you fast track your results. To learn more, go to:

https://www.cathymorenzie.com/coach

Share with Your Friends/Coworkers/Church

To order bulk copies of The Breakthrough Method, or any of Cathy's books, please contact support@weightlossgodsway.com

About The Author

Cathy Morenzie is CEO of and operates a min-
istry-minded health and weight-releasing com-
pany (weightlossgodsway.com) that has blessed
hundreds of thousands of women around the
world. She has been a voice to the faith based
health movement for over 35 years. She resides in
Barrie, Ontario, Canada with her family.

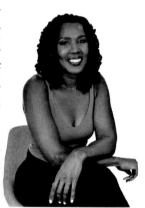

Cathy is a highly sought-after international
speaker and coach. She has given away 1 million
free teachings through YouVersion devotionals
and daily messages on YouTube.

Learn more at: cathymorenzie.com.

Follow Cathy at:

facebook.com/weightlossgodsway/

youtube.com/@CathyMorenzieWeightLossGodsWay

pinterest.com/cathymorenzie/

instagram.com/cathy.morenzie

Photos of Cathy Morenzie (both about the author & back cover images),
Deborah Lehman, Stephanie Franklin-Suber and Laura Foster by Val Westo-
ver Virtual Photography valwestoverphotography.com